"*The Psychosis Workbook* presents a comprehensive yet understandable explanation of psychosis. The authors have taken the mystery and fear out of the experience of psychosis, and replaced those with a clear and rational approach to help professionals understand the experience and those living with psychosis chart a path forward to health. *The Psychosis Workbook* is exceptionally clear, helpful, and complete. It should be required reading for all mental health clinicians."

> —**Mary A. Jansen, PhD**, former chair of the American Psychological Association (APA) Task Force on Serious Mental Illness and Severe Emotional Disturbance (TFSMI/SED), and vice president of the American Board of Serious Mental Illness and Severe Emotional Disturbance

"Although many textbooks and manuals have been written about psychosocial approaches for psychosis, there are few workbooks that are written directly for individuals with psychosis. This workbook offers a clear, accessible, and comprehensive approach to support individuals to draw upon a range of therapy approaches to enhance their own healing and recovery."

> —**Kate Hardy, ClinPsychD**, clinical professor in the INSPIRE Clinic at Stanford University, director of INSPIRE Training, and coeditor of *Decoding Delusions*

"A wonderfully comprehensive, well-researched, and non-stigmatizing guide to helping yourself with any form of psychosis. A truly person-centered and humanizing tool that fills a wide void in the market. As a psychosis community advocate and stabilized schizophrenic myself, I would recommend *The Psychosis Workbook* to anyone looking for support with their symptoms."

> —**Rose Parker**, schizophrenia and psychosis advocate and educator, and @PsychosisPsositivity author

"Supporting the development of the skills and attitudes necessary to achieve personal goals and manage distress is essential to helping individuals living with psychosis create rich, full lives. Either used for self-help or as a therapy companion, this long-overdue workbook offers a comprehensive, hopeful set of accessible tools to help individuals living with psychosis build lives worth living. There is nothing else like this out there."

> —**Shirley M. Glynn, PhD, ABSMIP**, research psychologist at UCLA, licensed psychologist with a private practice in Southern California, and coauthor of *Behavioral Family Therapy for Serious Psychiatric Illnesses*

"*The Psychosis Workbook* is a much-needed resource for people with mental illnesses. The authors use clear, straightforward language to demystify the experiences associated with psychosis, and provide a wealth of resources, skills, and exercises that will help those with psychosis successfully manage their symptoms and start their path toward recovery. Empowering and hopeful, this workbook will change people's lives for the better."

> —**Jennifer Snyder, PhD**, associate chief of psychology at Oregon State Hospital; and past president of APA Division 18: Psychologists in Public Service

"This book is chock-full of practical information and advice, ranging from understanding the nature of psychosis to developing a plan to stay well, coping with common symptoms, and preventing relapses. The guide is easy to use, replete with numerous worksheets and engaging and inspiring vignettes, all written in clear, nontechnical, and recovery-oriented language. This is an essential tool for anyone seeking to regain control over their lives after experiencing psychosis."

> —**Kim T. Mueser, PhD**, professor of occupational therapy and psychological and brain sciences, and former executive director of the Center for Psychiatric Rehabilitation at Boston University

"*The Psychosis Workbook* is a breath of fresh air for the recovery movement, a zephyr which can help lift families and loved ones with psychosis out of pessimistic stagnation and into a meaningful recovery trajectory. I strongly endorse this volume and will be recommending it during my international webinars and workshops on cognitive behavioral therapy (CBT) for psychosis."

> —**Douglas Turkington, MD**, professor of psychiatry at Newcastle University in the UK, and coauthor of *Treating Psychosis*

The Psychosis Workbook

Understand What You're Going Through, Take an Active Role in Your Recovery, and Prevent Relapse

LAURA DEWHIRST, PSYD
JESSICA MURAKAMI-BRUNDAGE, PHD

New Harbinger Publications, Inc.

Copyright © 2024 by Laura Dewhirst and Jessica Murakami-Brundage
New Harbinger Publications, Inc.
5720 Shattuck Avenue
Oakland, CA 94609
www.newharbinger.com

Cover design by Amy Shoup

Acquired by Jennye Garibaldi

Edited by Gretel Hakanson

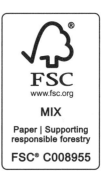

Printed in the United States of America

26   25   24

10   9   8   7   6   5   4   3   2   1   First Printing

To those of you who allowed me into your struggles and triumphs with psychosis. You were the inspiration and ongoing motivation for this project.

—LD

To the residents at the Oregon State Hospital, who struggle and overcome tremendous obstacles every single day.

—JMB

Contents

Foreword

Rufus May currently works as a psychologist helping people with psychosis, but when he was eighteen, it was he who became paranoid and was diagnosed with schizophrenia. Professionals at the time explained what they thought had gone wrong with his mind, but he noticed that the way they framed things made him feel like the passive victim of an active illness, with no room for hope that his own efforts could lead to recovery.

Fortunately, Rufus later met others who were more encouraging, and he found ways to regain control of his life and to move toward a meaningful future.

People shouldn't have to be lucky, however, to hear about active approaches to recovery from psychosis: such ideas should be available to everyone! This workbook is a great step in that direction.

I first met one of the authors, Jessica Murakami-Brundage, when she was an intern assisting me in facilitating a hearing voices group. I've taught a multitude of students, but Jessica stands out as someone who was subsequently inspired to learn and work with leaders in the field and who is now, with this publication coauthored by her own former student Laura Dewhirst, stepping into leadership herself.

When a path is well laid out, it seems simple and easy to follow. So it is with the exercises in this workbook. But those familiar with the variety of often conflicting therapy approaches for psychosis will recognize that impressive work was done to boil down the wisdom of those various modalities into this very user-friendly format.

Better yet, the authors have done so in a way that is not superficial. They offer creative approaches even for some of the deeper and trickier issues, such as exercises exploring the possible meaning behind what a voice is saying and guidance in how to respond to a voice in a way that balances assertiveness with compassion toward both the voice hearer and the voice.

Still though you may be asking, "How much can a workbook do to help someone escape from something as daunting as psychosis?"

One way of understanding psychosis is as something that results when our minds experiment with seeing things differently, and then get lost somewhere, or tangled up. Once this occurs, it's easy for us to lose confidence in ourselves. How can we possibly use that same mind to get us out of a trap that it has created?

We might recall the wise saying that "if you are going through hell, keep going!" Our minds may have gotten us into a confused or hellish place, but stopping mental experimentation can be an unhelpful solution, sort of like stopping in hell. A better approach might be to recognize that while we've wandered into making sense of things in a way that doesn't work very well, we can keep experimenting with other ways of making sense until we find something that works better.

That's what this workbook is about: experimenting with possibly better ways of making sense. The authors provide some ways of understanding psychotic experiences, but they also acknowledge that the perspectives they offer are not the only possibilities. That's important because there are many unresolved questions not only about psychosis but also about the nature of reality itself. What people need is not a one-size-fits-all view but help in finding a perspective that fits them personally and facilitates forming good relationships with others and creating a meaningful life.

Another barrier to recovery can be the exaggerated negative views of people with psychosis held by many professionals and members of the public. Such "stigma" can then be internalized by the person with psychosis, causing huge problems. Oryx Cohen has stated that after he first became psychotic, the way psychosis and its implications were explained to him made him feel as if he was being kicked out of the human race! Fortunately, he later found better ways to understand what was happening, and he now helps others recover through his work as chief executive officer of the National Empowerment Center. Escaping from stigma is not easy, and some have reported it can be more difficult than dealing with psychosis itself, but the exercises in this workbook on resisting stigma and discrimination can help people begin to break free.

The journey of a thousand miles truly does begin with a single step. I'm hoping that you will find that this workbook facilitates some very significant early steps in your journey toward recovery and toward fashioning the life you want.

—Ron Unger, LCSW
https://recoveryfrompsychosis.org

Welcome Letter

Thank you for picking up this workbook and being here. Being told that you have "psychosis" can provoke many thoughts and emotions. On one hand, you may feel comforted that there is a name for what you are experiencing. On the other hand, you may feel overwhelmed, confused as to why it's happening, or scared about what it means for your future. You may also disagree with this label.

While your thoughts and feelings about psychosis will likely change over time, an important thing to remember is that *you are not alone.* In fact, it is estimated that psychosis impacts three to six out of every one hundred people in their lifetime, and one hundred thousand new young people in the United States each year (McGrath et al. 2015; NAMI 2024). Although psychosis is most often associated with a diagnosis of a "schizophrenia spectrum and other psychotic disorder," including schizophrenia, schizoaffective disorder, and delusional disorder, psychosis itself can occur within over forty psychiatric and medical diagnoses—or may not be associated with any kind of diagnosis. It may also accompany several temporary states, such as bereavement and sensory deprivation.

In fact, we are all capable of experiencing psychosis under the right conditions. It is part of the incredible spectrum of experiences that are possible for us to encounter as human beings. People have been hearing voices and experiencing visions for millennia. In some cultures, what we now call "psychosis" is considered a spiritual gift of great value. Indeed, psychosis has been associated with enhanced creativity and thought to serve an evolutionary purpose—as a way for humans to take great leaps in thinking, pushing our society forward by helping us think of things in new ways (Barrantes-Vidal 2004; Turkington et al. 2009).

However, the positive aspects of psychosis are often overshadowed by how incredibly disruptive psychosis can be. Treatment can often greatly reduce this disruption, yet only about 29 percent of people who experience psychosis receive mental health treatment (World Health Organization 2022). For those who receive help, it takes seventy-two weeks (almost a year and a half!), on average, from the onset of psychosis for treatment to begin (NAMI 2024). We strongly believe that effective treatments and strategies for coping with psychosis should be available to everyone who wants them—that is why we worked together to write this workbook.

In these ten chapters, we will offer you a diverse range of interventions for psychosis drawn from several different therapies that have been shown to be effective in the treatment of psychosis in conjunction with medication. Research has consistently demonstrated that a combination of medication and therapy is almost always more effective than medication alone (Guo et al. 2010; Hogarty and Ulrich 1998; Menditto et al. 1996; Mojtabai et al. 1998). The interventions we draw from include cognitive behavioral therapy (CBT, often referred to as cognitive behavioral therapy for psychosis, or CBTp, when applied to psychosis), acceptance and commitment therapy (ACT), dialectical behavioral therapy (DBT), cognitive remediation therapy (CRT), and compassion-focused therapy (CFT).

We want to assure you that although your experience of psychosis may be highly emotional and deeply personal, there are ways to manage and ultimately recover from psychosis. Here "recovery" refers to living a rich and meaningful life, despite or even because of symptoms of psychosis. If you have ever felt as if your symptoms are interfering with your ability to find peace, feel good about yourself, build relationships, or achieve your goals, then this book is for you. We encourage you to start at the beginning and read every chapter even if you think it may not apply to your experience, as the skills complement and build on one another. In addition to symptoms of psychosis, we also cover related topics and experiences, such as depression, suicidal ideation, and stigma.

Between the two of us, we have over twenty-five years of experience working with people with psychosis. We have been fortunate to have been part of this process for hundreds of people who have struggled with psychosis and are extremely grateful to hopefully be part of this process for you too. We encourage you to share this workbook with the people you trust as you try out these strategies and make sense of your experiences. We have included copies of many of the exercises found in this workbook on the website for this book, http://www.newharbinger.com/53394, so you can do them more than once. There, you will also find bonus tools and resources for psychosis, including a list of websites and books we recommend. Working with a therapist may also deepen your understanding of these topics and how to apply these skills.

Let's get started!

Warmly,
Laura and Jessica

CHAPTER 1.

What Is Psychosis?

When we ask our clients to describe their earliest memory of experiencing psychosis, oftentimes they will begin by sharing, "I noticed *something felt different*."

Some describe first noticing changes to their mood or energy levels, such as feeling more anxious or energized than usual. Others describe a change to how they were thinking about things, such as worrying that other people were upset with them or noticing an onslaught of new and exciting ideas. More still describe noticing changes to how their mind worked, for example, feeling mentally "foggy," noticing things in their environment appeared slightly distorted, seeing shadows out of the corners of their eyes, or hearing voices that were difficult to locate.

There is no one answer because *there is no one way to experience psychosis*. Instead, psychosis is a highly diverse and deeply personal experience, one that is influenced by several factors, including your environment and personal history.

We begin this book by offering you important information on psychosis. Learning more about psychosis is a crucial part of your recovery; by better understanding what is happening, you can reassure yourself that there is a name for what you are experiencing, that you are not alone (many people experience psychosis), and that what you are experiencing is something that can be managed and overcome.

Here's how learning more about psychosis helped Rick feel more empowered in his recovery:

I usually know when I'm about to have an episode of psychosis. It's subtle, but I can feel the change happening. I remember when I had my first episode; one of the scariest parts was not understanding what was happening to me or why. Now that I've learned more about psychosis, I can often reassure myself that what I am going through is not as scary as it seems and get help faster if I need it.

Defining Psychosis

Psychosis is not one single thing. Instead, *psychosis* refers to some combination of the following: hallucinations, delusions, and changes to your behavior, mood, and cognition (for example, your ability to focus and organize your thoughts). Together, these changes result in a loss of touch with reality, making it hard to differentiate between what is real and not real, or false.

Below we will discuss each of the major symptoms of psychosis. We will then explore how these symptoms may impact your perception of reality. As you read, you may notice some of the sections do not fit with your personal experience—that is expected! Everyone's psychosis is different, and it is common for people to have some symptoms more than others.

New or Amplified Experiences: The "Positive" Symptoms

For some, psychosis is an experience characterized by a surge of new thoughts and perceptions. These are sometimes called the *positive symptoms* of psychosis, and include hallucinations, delusions, and changes in behavior.

In this context, "positive" means in addition to, which refers to how these experiences can feel like an amplification of your inner world. It is not uncommon for these experiences to be described as overwhelming, disorienting, or distracting.

Hallucinations

Sometimes referred to as false perceptions, *hallucinations* are sensory phenomena in the absence of external stimuli. This includes things like hearing voices other people don't hear or seeing things others don't see. Hallucinations can feel and look just like non-hallucinatory perceptions—which is what makes them so convincing! Hallucinations may occur in any sensory modality (sight, sound, smell, taste, touch). Auditory hallucinations are the most common type of hallucination associated with the diagnoses of schizophrenia and schizoaffective disorders (Compton and Broussard 2009). Because hallucinations of all types are fairly common, the presence of hallucinations alone is not sufficient for a diagnosis of a psychiatric or medical condition.

Here is Lynn's description of her hallucinations:

I hear voices daily. The first time I heard a voice, I felt startled—I tried to find out where it was coming from, but it never seemed to be coming from anywhere in particular. The more I heard the voices, the more comfortable I got with them. Sometimes I'll also feel things on my skin—almost like someone is pinching me or something is crawling on me. When those started, they really panicked me. I still don't like them, but now I have a lot of practice reassuring myself that I am safe, and I am able to redirect my attention to something else.

Below is a list of other common hallucinatory experiences reported by others. Check off any you have had or write in your own:

- ☐ Hearing voices or whispers when no one is there

- ☐ Hearing sounds (for example, electronic, buzzing, mechanical, or animal noises) without a known source

- ☐ Feeling things on my skin, such as zaps, tingling sensations, or feeling like something is crawling on me

- ☐ Feeling as if my body or organs are being squeezed, moved, or altered

- ☐ Seeing flashes of light, spots, or lines

- ☐ Seeing shadows

- ☐ Seeing colors change

- ☐ Seeing "glitches"

- ☐ Seeing faces change or noticing people I know look unlike themselves

- ☐ Tasting things I have not eaten or drank

- ☐ Smelling things other people do not, such as a gas leak or a rotten or sulfurous smell

- ☐ Write your own: _____

- ☐ Write your own: _____

Building Awareness: Do you experience hallucinations, such as hearing voices? If so, how have these experiences impacted your life?

_____

_____

_____

_____

_____

_____

_____

_____

Delusions

Psychosis can impact your beliefs in addition to your perceptions. *Delusions* refer to beliefs that are not true but seem to *feel* true. These beliefs, by nature, persist even after you have seen evidence that directly contradicts them. Delusional beliefs can be incredibly difficult to ignore, especially if they are frightening or are related to your safety. A key feature of delusions is that they are not typically shared by others in your culture. For example, some people believe that they are dead, despite the fact that they are breathing and talking. This is an unusual belief that does not match the facts and is not shared by others.

Consider Lesia's story, which highlights how her hallucinations contributed to the development of her delusion that she was God:

> Last spring was the first time my energy changed. It felt like a rush, like an internal intensity I had never felt before. I was sleeping less but wasn't tired—I was able to accomplish so much, no longer bogged down by my depression. I had all these ideas for new creative projects and felt deeply connected to my environment. I began hearing a voice that told me I was powerful and all-knowing and that all the new ideas I was having

would help humanity. I eventually came to the conclusion that the voice must be an angel—and that I was God. I felt responsible for all humankind. Watching the news made the voice louder. Any time there was any type of tragedy or a natural disaster, I felt personally responsible—the voice would turn on me and tell me how horrible I was and how it was my fault things were going wrong. I felt so guilty and would spend hours isolating myself so I could direct my energy outward to the people who needed my help.

Below are some other common delusions. Note that these are only delusions if they are, in fact, not true (if you are unsure, that's okay; we will spend more time exploring this topic in chapter 5). Check off the beliefs you currently have or have had in the past that others disagreed with:

- ☐ *I am a religious figure.*

- ☐ *I am a celebrity.*

- ☐ *I have a powerful role or job.*

- ☐ *I am very rich.*

- ☐ *Someone famous, or someone I have had little contact with, is in love with me.*

- ☐ *I have an illness or am pregnant when repeated medical tests say otherwise.*

- ☐ *Something has been inserted in my body or is living in my body.*

- ☐ *People are out to get me.*

- ☐ *I am being tracked, watched, or monitored.*

- ☐ *There is a conspiracy against me.*

- ☐ *Other people are talking about me.*

- ☐ *There are hidden messages for me in my environment.*

- ☐ Write your own: _____

- ☐ Write your own: _____

Building Awareness: If you checked any of the beliefs on the previous page, write down how these beliefs have impacted your life in the space below.

_____

_____

_____

_____

_____

_____

_____

_____

Reduced Feelings and Experiences: The "Negative" Symptoms

"Negative" symptoms of psychosis include feeling less motivated, less enthusiastic, less able to experience your emotions, or speaking less than you usually would. In this context, "negative" refers to having something taken away, or reduced.

Below are common negative symptoms of psychosis. Check off any you have noticed in your experience, or write in your own:

☐ *I have less to say.*

☐ *I smile and laugh less.*

☐ *I feel numb.*

☐ *I do not get out of bed much.*

☐ *I feel slow or move less.*

☐ *It feels hard or impossible to feel happy.*

☐ *I have a hard time eating.*

☐ *I have a hard time taking care of myself.*

☐ *I feel apathetic or disinterested in things I used to enjoy.*

☐ *I have no motivation to do anything.*

☐ Write your own: _____

☐ Write your own: _____

Building Awareness: Some people report that their negative symptoms, such as loss of motivation, help protect them from how overwhelming their positive symptoms, such as paranoia, feel. Sometimes these symptoms can result from medication side effects. If you experience negative symptoms, do you have an explanation for them, and if so, what is your explanation?

_____

_____

_____

_____

_____

_____

_____

Changes in Your Thinking—The Cognitive Symptoms

Cognitive symptoms refer to changes in how your mind works—including how it processes and organizes information—and how you are able to communicate with others. Common cognitive symptoms of psychosis include having trouble focusing, planning, or problem solving and jumbling up your words when you talk.

Below are some other common cognitive symptoms of psychosis. Check off any you have noticed in your experience or write in your own:

☐ I have trouble concentrating or focusing on activities.

☐ It's hard to learn new things.

☐ It's hard to remember things.

☐ It's difficult to make a plan or organize things.

☐ Tasks feel more difficult than usual.

☐ It's hard to focus on a single thought.

☐ I feel worn out by long or tedious tasks.

☐ It's hard to pay attention when people are talking to me.

☐ It's hard to know if people are joking or not.

☐ I feel like I don't really understand what people are talking about.

☐ It's hard to understand sarcasm, proverbs, or colloquial phrases, like "An apple a day keeps the doctor away," or "Cost me an arm or a leg."

☐ My words feel jumbled, or people tell me they are having trouble following what I am saying.

☐ I use words incorrectly or say words that don't exist.

☐ Write your own: _____

☐ Write your own: _____

Building Awareness: Have you experienced any cognitive changes since the onset of your psychosis or even preceding your psychosis? If so, how has this impacted you?

_____

_____

_____

_____

_____

Changes in Your Feelings, Thinking, and Behavior

Together, the positive, negative, and cognitive symptoms of psychosis impact how you feel, how you think, and what you do. In particular, others may notice changes in your behavior. Check off those that apply to you:

☐ Changes to how you dress or groom yourself

☐ Feeling excessively restless or spending a lot of time walking or pacing

☐ Isolating more or lying in bed more

☐ Eating less or not at all

☐ Engaging in repetitive behaviors, such as repeatedly touching something, walking in circles, or repeatedly doing an activity (for example, turning on the microwave or moving objects about the room)

☐ Doing things that jeopardize your safety, such as walking into traffic or going outside on a freezing day without a jacket

Some behavioral changes stem from how distracting and consuming other symptoms of psychosis can be. For example, it is hard to pay attention to what is going on around you when you are hearing loud or distressing voices. Other times, your behaviors may change because you are doing something *in response* to a hallucination or delusion, for example, going outside without a jacket because a voice told you to or throwing away your food because you suspect it might be poisoned.

Building Awareness: Do any of your behaviors change when you experience psychosis? Describe what you notice.

_____

_____

_____

_____

_____

How Psychosis Impacts Your Reality

The combined result of the many features of psychosis is a loss of touch with reality. In other words, during an episode of psychosis, some of the beliefs you hold, the conclusions you draw, or how you interpret the intentions of others will be biased, or heavily influenced, by the symptoms you are experiencing.

For example, let's imagine you begin to feel very unlike yourself or have the sense that something is wrong, but you are not sure what (these are early symptoms of psychosis). You then begin hearing voices when you're in conversations with others telling you, "They're lying," or "Watch out." You also begin noticing strange sensations in your body. In this state, you find yourself increasingly suspicious of the intentions of others. This leads you to the conclusion, *My food has been poisoned*—a terrifying thought for sure. But is it true? Or is it false, and instead only *feels true* in the context of your psychosis?

In this case, it would be possible to determine if your belief is true or not by having your food tested in a lab or by having a willing participant eat it and seeing what happens to them. Now let's say you tested your food, and the test revealed it was safe to eat. If you continue to believe that your food has been poisoned no matter what the evidence, then there is a difference between your *subjective reality* and your *objective reality*. Here, subjective reality refers to a perspective based on feelings, opinions, and emotions, while objective reality refers to a perspective based on facts and evidence (also what most others would consider to be true).

In many cases, false conclusions, such as the example above or the delusions listed earlier, continue to persist during an episode of psychosis because they *feel very true* to the person experiencing psychosis. This can be personally devastating if false conclusions keep you in a state of chronic fear or lead you to do things that jeopardize your safety.

The Hearing Voices Network, a worldwide community of people who offer support for people who hear voices, see visions, or experience other unusual perceptions, makes the distinction between "nonconsensus reality," your private experience of reality (such as the example above, the persistent belief that your food has been poisoned despite evidence disputing that conclusion) and "consensus reality," the reality that has been decided on by the person's larger group or society. Such a distinction recognizes how our realities are socially constructed (determined by our larger society).

The nature of reality is a complicated subject and beyond the scope of this workbook—and our knowledge. However, we offer a definition of psychosis that assumes that there is a subjective reality and an objective reality and that we can be right or wrong about something. Later, you'll learn how to test these beliefs and challenge thoughts or experiences that negatively impact your quality of life. While this may be considered a simplistic approach, we believe it is a practical one that lends itself to learning how to best function in our shared world.

What Causes Psychosis, and How Is It Treated?

Advancements in science have helped us identify our genes, life experiences, and neurochemistry as important contributors in creating psychotic experiences. While there is no one cause, below are some of the better understood risk factors for psychosis:

Psychosis Runs in the Family

Psychotic spectrum disorders, such as schizophrenia, are now understood to be highly hereditary, meaning you are more likely to develop psychosis if you are closely related to someone who also has experienced it (Compton and Broussard 2009). Take a moment to think about your family. Are there any members who also experience episodes of psychosis or have a diagnosis of schizophrenia, schizoaffective, or bipolar disorder?

How Stress and Trauma Contribute to Psychosis

Our brains change in response to stress. *Acute stress*, such as the sudden death of a loved one, a natural disaster, or a history of childhood or adult trauma, and *chronic stress*, such as social adversity (for example, racism, poverty, discrimination) have both been implicated in the development of psychosis (Turkington and Spencer 2019).

Consider Mateo's experience of how a history of childhood trauma contributed to his psychosis:

I was sexually abused by my mom's boyfriend when I was six. It happened a few times before they eventually broke up. When it was happening, he would tell me, "You're going to be in big trouble if anyone ever finds out about this. Your mom is going to be really mad at you." I didn't know what to do. I was so stressed whenever he was at the house, even if nothing ended up happening. After they broke up, I still worried my mother would find out. Eventually I worried everyone would find out and judge me for what had happened to me. I thought the worst of myself and other people. I began to hear voices telling me I was gay and that I was a bad person. The sound of other people laughing was so painful and humiliating, even when my friends would reassure me no one was laughing at me.

Building Awareness: Think back to your first episode of psychosis. Can you identify any areas of significant stress or change that occurred around that time? List them below. How might these experiences have impacted your psychosis?

_____

_____

_____

_____

_____

_____

_____

_____

Psychosis as a Result of Substance Use

Just as stress and trauma change our brains, taking drugs and alcohol changes our brains as well. While some substances are known to cause transitory symptoms of psychosis, such as LSD, the following drugs may cause *long-term symptoms* of psychosis, meaning the symptoms of psychosis could persist even after the initial effects of the substance have worn off:

- Stimulants, including methamphetamine, cocaine, and crack, and the abuse of prescribed stimulants, such as Adderall

- Cannabis, specifically if (1) use begins in childhood or adolescence when the brain is still developing, and (2) you have a genetic predisposition or early-life risk factors for psychosis (Compton and Broussard 2009)

- Inhalants (such as paint thinner, gasoline, kerosene, acetone, ether)

With these drugs, symptoms of psychosis can sometimes last for weeks or months following discontinuing use.

Building Awareness: Many people use drugs to move away from an unpleasant feeling, for example, to decrease boredom, feel more comfortable in social situations, try something exciting, or relax. If you use drugs or alcohol, do you notice you use them to avoid unpleasant feelings? Can you identify these feelings here?

_____

_____

Psychosis and Pregnancy

Biological females have higher rates of mood-congruent psychosis (when psychosis only occurs during an episode of depression or mania) and hormone-related psychosis, including postpartum psychosis and psychosis stemming from thyroid disease (Blake et al. 2015).

The onset for postpartum psychosis, or psychosis after the birth of a baby, is typically within the first two weeks after a woman has given birth. Risk factors for postpartum psychosis include new or worsening sleep deprivation, medical complications during pregnancy or birth, a family history of psychosis, and increased stress (Bennett and Indman 2019). *Postpartum psychosis should be considered an emergency*, as mother and baby are both highly vulnerable in the days and months after birth. It is recommended a medical professional be consulted as soon as symptoms of postpartum psychosis are suspected.

What Is Happening in the Brain

Our understanding of how our neurochemistry impacts our moods and mental health has come a long way in the last century and only continues to improve. By studying the brain, we have been able to better understand what kinds of changes the brain undergoes during an episode of psychosis. However, there is still much that is unknown. Below are some of the neurotransmitters that have been implicated in psychosis (neurotransmitters transmit messages from one nerve cell to the next in your nervous system—your nervous system controls everything from breathing and movement to senses and emotions):

- The neurotransmitter *dopamine* plays many important roles in the brain, including helping with mood, sleep, movement, pleasure, and memory. If you experience psychosis, you may have higher levels of dopamine in some parts of the brain and lower levels of dopamine in other parts (Compton and Broussard 2009).

- Changes to the neurotransmitters *glutamate*, GABA, and *serotonin* have also been observed in psychosis, with decreased glutamate activity potentially explaining some of the negative and cognitive symptoms of psychosis (Compton and Broussard 2009; Spaulding, Silverstein, and Menditto 2017).

How Do Medications Help?

In short, psychiatric medications work by acting on your neurotransmitters (messengers in the brain). This is the reason some people refer to mental health conditions as "chemical imbalances"—they're referring to the "balance" of your neurotransmitters. However, research into the causes of mental illness have not supported a "chemical imbalance theory," and it is largely considered to be overly simplistic or incorrect. Although it is not completely clear why antipsychotic medications work, research shows that these medications help to eliminate or noticeably reduce the symptoms of psychosis for most people (Haddad and Correll 2018).

One way to think about medications is as a foundation to begin building on. For example, if psychosis has disrupted your life in such a way that it has made it difficult or impossible to attend therapy, keep a job, finish school, or build a relationship, medication may be able to reduce symptoms enough so you can begin working on these goals. However, medications also tend to come with a lot of side effects that can be difficult to manage. It is important to work with your psychiatric provider to weigh the costs and benefits of medications and find what works the best for you. The goal is to maximize the benefits and minimize the side effects of medication. If you have questions about medications, schedule a time to meet with a psychiatric provider because they specialize in treating psychosis with medications.

Building Awareness: What are your thoughts about taking medications? If you already take medications for psychosis, how have they worked for you? What, if anything, would you change about them?

_____

_____

_____

_____

_____

_____

_____

_____

_____

_____

The remainder of this workbook will focus on psychological treatments for psychosis. Psychological interventions are one of many psychosocial treatments for psychosis; other psychosocial treatments include vocational rehabilitation, supported education, spiritual services, occupational therapy, recreation therapy, culturally specific services, and peer-led services. We hope such services are readily available to you and that you have one of the most important components of recovery: choice. Moving forward, we will offer you several skills to choose from that we have learned through our field of study. Find what works for you. Just as your experience of psychosis is unique to you, so are the assortment of skills that you find to be the most helpful.

Summary

Psychosis is a diverse experience, and no two people's psychosis is the same. However, there are several key features of psychosis that can help you identify when you are experiencing it, including hallucinations, delusions, and changes to your feelings, thinking, and behavior. Treatments for psychosis include medications and psychosocial interventions, including psychological interventions, such as the ones covered in this workbook. An important first step is identifying your strengths, values, and goals. This is the focus of the next chapter and will help give you some direction for the journey that lies ahead!

CHAPTER 2.

Your Recovery Road Map

Now that you have a better understanding of what psychosis is, your next step is to create a road map for recovery. First, however, let's talk about what it means to recover from psychosis.

In the past, people with psychosis, especially those diagnosed with schizophrenia, were thought to have a lifelong and worsening course of illness over time (Kendler 2020). We now know, however, that this is incorrect, as shown in Betram's case:

> During my first hospitalization, I was diagnosed with schizophrenia and told that I would never have a full-time job. Fortunately, I never believed them. I accepted their help—I took meds and applied for social security. I was discharged and eventually started working at the mall part time. Those first few years were really rough. Eventually, I went back to school to become a computer programmer. Now, I have a master's degree and work full-time.

Unfortunately, pessimism about the chances of recovery from psychosis remains in the mental health field—perhaps you have encountered this. It is important to remember that *the majority of people who experience psychosis will recover from it, either partially or completely, with symptoms decreasing over time* (Jeblensky et al. 1992).

Even if you have a diagnosis of what is considered a serious mental illness, such as severe major depression, bipolar disorder, or schizophrenia, that causes you to have difficulty functioning in at least one major area of your life (school, work, relationships, activities of daily living), your symptoms are likely to improve over time and become easier to manage.

However, recovery has come to mean so much more than symptom reduction. The *recovery model* of mental illness recognizes that *everyone* who experiences psychosis is capable of leading full and meaningful lives (Bellack and Drapalski 2012). Your recovery is a process of learning about yourself, reaching your goals, and living a full life either with or despite symptoms of mental illness. It does not require the elimination of your symptoms. Indeed, the goal of this workbook is not to help you get rid of symptoms, but to help you learn how to live the life that you want without your symptoms interfering. You may also find your psychotic experiences to be a source of meaning.

In this chapter, we will delve more into what recovery means to you: What does it mean to reach your full potential? What do you want your life to look like? What is important to you? Your recovery journey is uniquely your own. You are the hero of your journey, the main character of your own unfolding story. We don't know the unique challenges you face, but we believe that you can benefit from some of the same skills and tools that others have benefitted from and that have been shown to be effective. The recovery road map you will complete in this chapter will help guide you on your journey, reminding you of the skills you can practice when any obstacle arises and providing you with an overall sense of direction. We welcome you to return to your road map again and again, tracking your progress and making updates as you go.

Remember that you are a complex human being filled with tremendous possibilities—you cannot be defined by labels or symptoms of mental illness. We fully believe that you can, and will be able to, overcome the challenges of psychosis with the right combination of knowledge, skills, resources, and support. This process of discovery and growth is truly a journey of recovery.

Building Awareness: How would you define recovery? What would lead you to say you were "recovered" from psychosis?

_____

_____

_____

_____

_____

_____

_____

Your Recovery Road Map

Let's turn our attention to creating your road map to recovery. The first part of this road map will be all about you and what you bring with you on your journey. Then, you will look at obstacles in your journey, tools to overcome these obstacles, and those who will accompany you. Take your time as you fill this out, and feel free to invite others who know you well to help you. Some sections may be easier than others—that's to be expected. Try your best to fill out every section of your road map. You will be able to add to each section as you go through the rest of the chapters, especially the tools section.

Part I. The Hero (You!)

Draw yourself in the space below. Around your drawing, list your various identities, including the roles you have in life that include duties and responsibilities (such as parent, child, sibling, friend, student) and groups that you identify with (such as veterans, ethnic, or racial groups).

PERSONAL STRENGTHS

What strengths do you bring with you on your journey? What do you like most about yourself? What do other people like about you? Think about the compliments you have received over the course of your life, even if you do not necessarily agree. What personal qualities have made it possible for you to overcome the challenges in your life so far? What kind of person are you? Are you kind, funny, strong, determined?

_____

_____

_____

_____

_____

_____

_____

_____

_____

_____

SKILLS AND TALENTS

What skills do you have? What talents do you possess? Perhaps you are a good listener or you are good at telling jokes. What are you good at? Is there anything you have gotten better at over time? Perhaps you are good at solving puzzles, singing, or noticing things in your environment that other people don't. List your skills and talents below.

_____

_____

_____

_____

_____

_____

_____

_____

_____

_____

RESOURCES

What material resources do you have available to you? These are resources that will help you on your recovery journey in your day-to-day life (for example, funds, housing, social security benefits, means of transportation, a cell phone). Resources also include your access to treatment, including a psychosocial rehabilitation program or a substance abuse treatment center.

_____

_____

_____

_____

_____

_____

_____

What immaterial resources do you have available to you? Think about things that support you, that you cannot necessarily hold in your hands (such as faith in God, hope for the future, support of family members, and connection with nature).

_____

_____

_____

_____

_____

_____

_____

VALUES

Values are an important part of your recovery journey and are very helpful in defining your goals. Values are not goals. Goals can be set and achieved, and once they are achieved, we see them as finished or completed. Unlike goals, values have no end point. Instead, they are what motivate and guide us through life (Hayes et al. 2012). They provide us with direction and act as a compass, especially when we feel lost or confused. The following activities are meant to give you some idea of your values.

Think of someone you deeply admire. It could be someone in your life, a notable historical figure, a movie character, or not a person at all (for example, a spiritual being, or favorite pet).

Person or being you admire: _____

What is it that you admire about this person or being? _____

_____

_____

_____

_____

_____

_____

_____

_____

Below is a list of values. Circle the ones you care about the most. Then make a star next to your top five values.

Courage	Independence	Freedom	Passion
Humility	Kindness	Security	Power
Duty	Generosity	Openness	Fairness
Responsibility	Faith	Fun	Insight
Integrity	Compassion	Adventure	Safety
Loyalty	Discipline	Gratitude	Flexibility
Balance	Honesty	Connection	Harmony
Learning	Wisdom	Contribution	Cooperation
Knowledge	Happiness	Love	Strength
Creativity	Productivity	Restraint	Curiosity
Dedication	Patience	Boldness	Simplicity
Perseverance	Responsibility	Gentleness	_____
Growth	Peace	Resilience	_____

What is your psychosis about? Psychosis seems to often target what people care the most about. Do you care about your family? You may hear a voice threaten to harm your family. Do you care about being a good person? You may hear a voice tell you that you are a terrible person. Alternatively, you may hear voices or have beliefs about being an extremely important person, which could reflect the desire to be appreciated or respected. Write down what your voices say or beliefs that you have related to your psychosis. What values are being reflected?

_____

_____

_____

_____

_____

_____

_____

_____

_____

_____

Below are some writing exercises to further help you identify your values.

1. Think of what causes you the most pain. Is it betrayal? A traumatic experience? The loss of a loved one? Loneliness? Often, we feel pain when we experience an attack on our values or when we are not able to realize them. Your pain tells you what you care about. Write down two to three sources of suffering in your life.

    _____

    _____

    _____

    _____

    _____

2.   The eulogy exercise (Hayes et al. 2012): Write the eulogy you would want written about you—how do you want to be remembered? What would you want a loved one to say about you at your funeral?

_____

_____

_____

_____

_____

_____

_____

3.   The "miracle question" (Strong and Pyle 2009): If you had a magic wand to grant any wish you'd like, what would you wish for (besides more wishes)? How would your life be different?

_____

_____

_____

_____

_____

_____

_____

GOALS

Setting goals for yourself is a skill that can be developed over time. Sometimes when people are just starting out, they may have trouble identifying personal goals or find their goals are so vague they do not give them a clear starting point. For example, if your goal is "I want to feel better," that is an excellent goal! However, it is vague, so it's unclear when you've achieved this goal or when to set a new goal. A more clearly defined goal would be "I want to feel more confident in myself. Right now, I would rate my self-confidence as a 3 out of 10 with 10 being the highest. I'd like to be at a 7 most days."

Goal setting is important because it is motivating and gives you something to work toward. Goals are destinations on your recovery journey. We've come up with several goals below in different categories of wellness. You don't need to come up with this many! The different categories may help you think of goals that you want to work on.

Examples of recovery goals include:

Psychological:

- "I would like to decrease the frequency of my voices by 50 percent."

Emotional:

- "I would like to learn ways to cope with feelings of sadness so they do not overwhelm me."

Occupational and academic:

- "I would like to finish my college degree and find a job working with animals."

Intellectual and creative:

- "I would like to work on my creative writing five times a week."

Recreational:

- "I would like to join a community softball league."

Physical:

- "I would like to walk for thirty minutes before work each day."

Financial:

- "I would like to save up to buy a car; I will put aside 10 percent of my paycheck every other week to reach my goal."

Religious and spiritual:

- "I would like to feel more connected to my higher power."

- "I would like to practice meditation at least three times a week."

Social:

- "I would like to reach out to my friends and family on a weekly basis."

- "I would like to get better at communicating my needs to my loved ones."

Community:

- "I would like to find at least one space in my community that feels welcoming."

- "I am interested in volunteering at my local food bank."

Try to think of goals that are SMART, as in specific, measurable, attainable, realistic, and time-bound (Doran 1981). This will make them easier to track and achieve, building confidence and motivating you to set new goals. We recommend setting both short, medium, and long-term goals.

Short-term goals (to achieve within the next three months):

1. _____

2. _____

3. _____

4. _____

5. _____

Medium-term goals (to achieve after three months and within the next year):

1. _____

2. _____

3. _____

4. _____

5. _____

Long-term goals (to achieve after one year and beyond):

1. _____

2. _____

3. _____

4. _____

5. _____

Part II. Obstacles

What gets in the way of achieving your goals? Obstacles are an important part of every journey. Sometimes obstacles are easy to define and predict. At other times, they take us by surprise. If we can prepare for obstacles in advance, we will be more successful at overcoming them. Even when they are unexpected, however, we can still learn from them and prepare for them in the future.

SYMPTOMS

Symptoms of mental illness can make ordinary challenges extremely difficult. For example, feeling very depressed can make it difficult to get out of bed. Medication side effects can do the same. What are the symptoms that most bother you? You may want to refer to chapter 1 when filling this out. Try to be specific (for example, instead of writing "psychosis," write down what symptom of psychosis is most bothersome, like "hearing critical voices").

1. _____

2. _____

3. _____

4. _____

5. _____

PROBLEMATIC BEHAVIORS

Sometimes we do things that work against our goals. For example, we may want a romantic relationship but avoid meeting new people. We may turn to drugs or alcohol to feel better, only to end up losing all motivation to get fit and healthy. What are the behaviors that you do (or don't do) that interfere with your goals? You may want to revisit your goals and think about what gets in your way of achieving each particular goal.

1. _____

2. _____

3. _____

4. _____

5. _____

PSYCHOLOGICAL ROADBLOCKS

Roadblocks can be messages we tell ourselves that hold us back. They can be beliefs or attitudes that are understandable, but not entirely helpful. For example, caring too much about what other people think can prevent us from trying new things. Thinking, *It's not worth it*, is also a limiting belief. Other psychological roadblocks include low self-confidence, low motivation, and lack of trust in others. What are some of the psychological roadblocks that get in the way of achieving your goals?

1. _____

2. _____

3. _____

4. _____

5. _____

EXTERNAL OBSTACLES

External obstacles don't come from us, but from other people and our situations. They can be huge, like poverty, or smaller and more specific, like not having transportation. Try to come up with specific external obstacles that get in your way. The more specific the obstacle, the easier it is to problem solve and overcome. For example, "a broken mental health system" is a huge obstacle that is impossible for one person to overcome completely. "Finding a good therapist" is a lot more manageable.

1. _____

2. _____

3. _____

4. _____

5. _____

Part III. Tools

Now that you have identified the obstacles that get in your way, you can start to identify the resources and tools that you will use to overcome these obstacles. Some of the skills that you have available to you can be included in more than one category.

BIOLOGICAL

Medication, herbal supplements, acupuncture, transcranial magnetic stimulation—these are all biological tools that can aid in your recovery journey. We are defining biological tools as the tools that work directly through your central nervous system (composed of the brain, spinal cord, and neurons). What are the biological tools available for you to use (for example, types of medication and natural remedies, such as fish oil)?

1. _____

2. _____

3. _____

4. _____

5. _____

BEHAVIORAL

Behavioral tools are things that you do. They can include healthy routines (such as keeping a structured schedule, getting between seven and nine hours of sleep every night, taking medication every day at the same time) and specific actions, such as going to therapy, meeting with a peer specialist, exercising three times per week, and practicing relaxation techniques. Don't get too hung up on trying to figure out if a specific action falls into this category or into a different category. What is important is to include all the tools you have available to you in this section of your recovery road map.

1. _____

2. _____

3. _____

4. _____

5. _____

PSYCHOLOGICAL

What are some of the psychological tools and skills that you can use to overcome obstacles as they arise? Psychological tools involve the mind and how we think about things. We expect this category, especially, will grow over time as you obtain more skills, including the psychological skills in this workbook. Examples of psychological tools include mindfulness, "changing my thoughts and beliefs," and "accepting things I cannot change." Psychological tools can overlap with behavioral tools (technically, changing our thinking is something that we do, so it is a behavior).

1. _____

2. _____

3. _____

4. _____

5. _____

SPIRITUAL

Spiritual tools include anything that helps you feel more connected to a higher power or a larger universe. Prayer may be included here, in addition to activities such as meditation. Going to church may be a spiritual activity that is also a social activity. What supports your spiritual well-being? Maybe it is being in nature or following a certain diet.

1. _____

2. _____

3. _____

4. _____

5. _____

RECREATIONAL

Having fun and being creative is an important part of life. What are the things that you enjoy doing? What are your hobbies? These are the activities that may bring a smile to your face or fill you with a sense of accomplishment.

1. _____

2. _____

3. _____

4. _____

5. _____

SOCIAL

Social tools and skills are things that you do with other people. These are the skills that keep you connected to others. Talking on the phone, going to meet-ups, and having dinner with your family would all be included here. Social skills and activities are an important part of recovery.

1. _____

2. _____

3. _____

4. _____

5. _____

If any of the categories above are blank, they may be areas to focus on when goal setting. If, for example, you do not have social outlets, it may be that "increasing my social circle" is a good medium-term goal. Skills, tools, and resources will help you overcome obstacles on your journey. They are also a big part of creating a rich and meaningful life.

Part IV. Your Support System

Who can you count on to support you in your recovery journey? Every hero's journey includes company and support along the way! Social support is a fundamental need that is associated with physical and emotional well-being (Taylor 2011). Feeling connected to and supported by others also helps us reach and celebrate our goals! Supportive others provide us with both tangible and intangible resources. Humans really are social creatures who benefit from close relationships. Family, friends, treatment team members, pets… write down the names of those in your social support system and their relationship to you in the space below.

Name	Relationship

Jim's Road Map to Recovery

Jim was nineteen years old when he started to hear voices. They started commenting on his actions but soon became critical and harsh. Jim tried his best to ignore them and did not discuss what he was experiencing with his roommates. At first, he continued going to his college classes but could not pay attention. He stopped going out with his friends, stopped showering, and eventually stopped leaving his room. He was convinced that his roommates were laughing at him and planning to harm him. His voices mocked him incessantly. After not eating or sleeping for days, he could be heard yelling in his room. Jim's roommates called his parents out of concern for him. His parents came to his apartment and convinced him to go to the hospital, where he was hospitalized and diagnosed with unspecified schizophrenia spectrum disorder. Jim started taking medication and was discharged soon afterward. He moved back home with his parents and took a leave of absence from college.

Below is Jim's recovery road map.

Part I: The Hero: Jim

Strengths: Hardworking, good sense of humor, willing to accept help, generous person

Skills and talents: Decent cook, conversational Spanish

Resources: Food and housing, Community Mental Health Center, have a bus pass, applying for SSI

Values: Respect, integrity, kindness, perseverance

Goals: Finish college with a major in education, get a job as an educator, move out and live on my own, get fit

Part II: Obstacles

Symptoms: Voices make it hard to concentrate, trouble focusing, sometimes I have panic attacks

Problematic behaviors: Avoidance and procrastination

Psychological roadblocks: Fear of failure, self-doubt

External obstacles: Meds make me really tired and hungry (so I end up eating a lot and being sedentary), limited funds; parents are supportive but can sometimes be overprotective; stigma

Part III: Tools

Biological: 5 milligrams of Risperdal for psychosis, melatonin to help me sleep, as needed

Behavioral: Go to bed and wake up around the same time every day (very important!), go walking for at least twenty minutes a day, eat three meals a day, shower every day, and wear clean clothes

Psychological: Practice mindfulness with my voices, distraction can sometimes help, remind myself that I am more powerful than my voices, do things that I'm afraid of to build my confidence

Spiritual: Being out in nature makes me feel connected to the wider universe

Recreational: Listen to music, go to concerts, practice speaking Spanish

Social: Go to Hearing Voices Network group once a week, meet with peer counselor (Eric), call best friend (George) and hang out, go out to dinner with my parents once a week

Part IV: Support System

Supports: Parents, George, Eric, our family's two dogs (Finn and Ezra)—good walking buddies, Hearing Voices Network group

Jim was able to go back to college. At first, he went back part time. He was tired a lot and worked with his psychiatrist to reduce his medications so he had more energy. He also practiced a lot of mindfulness techniques and made sure to stick to a routine. As he started to feel better about himself, he started attending a Hearing Voices Network group, where he learned from others how to better deal with his voices. He also made sure to stay connected with his best friend and started to expand his social network. He was able to go back to school full time and graduate with his college degree. He started working as a substitute teacher and eventually was hired on as a fourth-grade teacher. His next goal is to travel to Spain.

Your Recovery Road Map

Part I. The Hero

Personal strengths: _____

_____

_____

_____

_____

Skills and talents: _____

_____

_____

_____

_____

Resources: _____

_____

_____

_____

_____

Values: _____

_____

_____

_____

_____

Short-term goals: _____

_____

_____

_____

_____

Medium-term goals: _____

_____

_____

_____

_____

Long-term goals: _____

_____

_____

_____

_____

Part II. Obstacles

Symptoms: _____

_____

_____

_____

_____

Problematic behaviors: _____

_____

_____

_____

_____

Psychological roadblocks: _____

_____

_____

_____

_____

External obstacles: _____

_____

_____

_____

_____

Part III. Tools

Biological: _____

_____

_____

_____

Behavioral: _____

_____

_____

_____

_____

Psychological: _____

_____

_____

_____

_____

Spiritual: _____

_____

_____

_____

_____

Recreational: _____

_____

_____

_____

_____

Social: _____

_____

_____

_____

_____

Part IV. Your Support System

Name	Relationship

Summary

Recovery can be defined as a process of learning about yourself and living a full life either with or beyond your symptoms of mental illness. In this chapter, you've created a preliminary road map to your recovery that includes your strengths, values, goals, obstacles, tools, and supports. Don't worry if some sections are blank. You can always fill them in as you go. You can download and print a road map template on the website for this book: http://www.newharbinger.com/53394. Indeed, this workbook is focused on adding to your tools! Don't forget that you are the hero on your own unique journey of recovery. Next, you will focus on building a foundation of wellness that will help you move forward on your journey.

CHAPTER 3.

Building a Foundation for Wellness

In this chapter, we discuss foundational building blocks for mental wellness. No matter where you are in your journey, you will be more effective at overcoming obstacles and reaching your goals if you take care of yourself and approach your journey with a growth mindset (a commitment to learning as you go). With this in mind, we have grouped several foundational skills and activities into the following three categories:

- Taking care of your body by adopting healthy habits

- Taking care of your mind by practicing mindfulness

- Taking care of your heart through self-compassion

We call these foundational building blocks because each one is critically important in assisting you on your recovery journey. A strong and healthy body ensures you have the energy and stamina to keep going. Mindfulness allows you to be more aware of yourself and what is happening around you—this helps you problem solve effectively and enjoy your journey one step at a time. Meanwhile, self-compassion fosters resilience and patience on your journey, so you can persist despite setbacks.

As you move through this chapter, we encourage you to create a daily routine that incorporates the ideas we discuss here. A daily routine will make it significantly easier to stay on track and ensure your needs are being met consistently. We have included a sample routine, a blank routine template, and tips for overcoming barriers you might encounter on the website for this workbook, http://www.newharbinger .com/53394, to get you started. Remember, taking small steps every day can lead to big changes in the future—you and your health are well worth these investments!

Taking Care of Your Body by Adopting Healthy Habits

The first foundational building block for mental wellness is healthy habits. This section focuses on nourishing your body by incorporating more movement in your day, improving your sleep, eating nutritious meals, taking medications as prescribed, avoiding drugs and alcohol, and decreasing your stress. Although it is common to hear physical health and mental health described separately, our bodies and minds are part of the same system. The health of one directly influences the health of the other. By taking care of your body, you will feel better and have more energy. Your symptoms will also decrease and be more manageable.

Our Bodies Crave Movement

Let's start by discussing the foundational need for movement. You may have heard that getting regular physical activity and finding opportunities to move during the day can help improve your mood and reduce symptoms of depression and anxiety—but did you know that increasing your physical activity has also been shown to decrease symptoms of psychosis (Firth et al. 2015; Firth et al. 2018; Hunter et al. 2015; US Department of Health and Human Services 2018)?

Specifically, Firth et al. (2015, 2018) found that participants who engaged in ninety minutes of moderate to vigorous (think, running or playing a sport) exercise per week reported noticing significantly less negative and cognitive symptoms of psychosis (this could look like feeling more engaged, motivated, and more mentally focused).

Incorporating more movement into your day will also help improve your sleep quality; this is important because poor sleep quality, as you will see in the next section, has been associated with an increase in hallucinations and suspicious thoughts (Brederoo et al. 2021; Freeman et al. 2010; Martinez et al. 2024).

So how can you incorporate more movement into your week? First, you'll need to identify what activities you might be interested in. Write some ideas for what you would like to do for physical activity. Examples include walking, yoga, running, boxing, bodyweight training (for example, pushups, crunches, planks), swimming, bicycling, or playing a sport.

_____

_____

_____

_____

_____

Next, identify when (time of day) and for how long you will commit to engaging in this activity. Be specific if you can. For example, "Every day after breakfast, I will take a fifteen-minute walk around my neighborhood." Remember, the goal is at least ninety minutes per week. This could be broken up into three 30-minute sessions, or six 15-minute sessions per week.

_____

_____

_____

The Restorative Power of Sleep

When we sleep, we are giving our brains time to recover from the day and prepare for what lies ahead tomorrow. Research examining the relationship between symptoms of psychosis and sleep found that poor sleep is associated with experiencing an increase in hallucinations and perceptual disturbances (Brederoo et al. 2021; Van der Tuin et al. 2023).

Insomnia, or experiencing poor sleep quality or not enough sleep at least three times a week for a period of three months or more, has been identified as one of the earliest warning signs that an acute episode of psychosis may be coming (Bordoloi and Ramtekkar 2018; Compton and Broussard 2009). Insomnia has also been associated with a two- to three-time increase in suspicious thoughts or feelings of paranoia (Freeman et al. 2010; Martinez et al. 2024). This means that a night of poor sleep can make you feel incredibly anxious, on edge, and hypervigilant the next day, even if nothing is going wrong.

For these reasons, we encourage you to prioritize improving and regulating your sleep as part of taking care of yourself. Below are some sleep hygiene strategies that can help you succeed.

- Having a regular bedtime that allows for at least seven hours of sleep per night is a great way to get your sleep on track. Write a good bedtime for yourself here:

_____

- Electronic screens (such as TV, phone, video games) have been found to disrupt the hormone melatonin, which is important for sleep (Vartanian et al. 2015). If you're in the habit of using electronics before bed to wind down, what could do instead to help improve your sleep?

_____

_____

_____

- A good sleep environment has few distractions, is dark, and is not too warm. What are some ways you could improve your sleep environment?

  _____

  _____

  _____

  _____

  _____

  _____

- Sometimes when we try to sleep, our mind keeps wandering. When this happens, try getting up and doing a relaxing activity until you notice you're feeling sleepy. Good activities for this can include practicing deep breathing, working on a puzzle, reassuring yourself, or reading a book.

- Nightmares can make it very difficult to achieve restful sleep. If you wake up from a nightmare, try practicing the deep breathing techniques we cover later in this chapter and the defusion techniques in chapter 5. These can help soothe your body and mind and get you back to sleep.

Healthy Eating

The field of nutritional psychiatry explores how the food we eat impacts our mood and brain health. In short, it impacts it very much! What we put in our bodies has a direct impact on our mood and energy levels. This is why it is important to do our best to nourish our bodies with foods that help us feel good.

The book *Eat to Beat Depression and Anxiety: Nourish Your Way to Better Mental Health in Six Weeks* by Dr. Drew Ramsey (2021) identifies a healthy brain diet as one that incorporates plenty of fruits, whole grains, healthy fats, vegetables, and fish.

To help ensure your dietary needs are being met consistently, try these suggestions:

- Create a shopping list for the week. Include healthy meal options as well as healthy snacks (such as avocados, apples, nuts, smoked salmon, berries).

- Schedule a set day and time to grocery shop each week.

- Set aside time to prepare meals at home.

Building Awareness: New to cooking? Identify someone or something (for example, a cookbook, YouTube, or a cooking show) that could help get you started.

_____

_____

_____

Taking Medications as Prescribed

Taking medications as prescribed is a critical component of many treatment plans, as missing doses or stopping medications without the supervision of your physician often leads to new or worsening symptoms of psychosis, also known as a _mental health relapse_ (Turkington and Spencer 2019). Here's how you can problem solve medication concerns to ensure you take your medications as prescribed.

Work with your provider. First, if you have questions about your medications, are noticing unpleasant side effects, or are interested in changing your dose, speak to your psychiatric provider. They will be able to recommend alternatives (if available) and help you navigate changing doses safely. Your pharmacist can also be a great resource for information.

Set reminders. If you sometimes forget a dose, try setting reminders. This can include leaving yourself a note on your bathroom mirror or nightstand, setting an alarm on your phone, or adding refill dates on your calendar. Try to schedule refills at least a few days in advance in case something comes up that prevents you from getting to your pharmacy. Do the same for any injectable medications that require an appointment.

Avoid the "but I'm feeling better" trap. It is extremely common for people to tell us they stopped taking their medications without talking to their physician first because _they were feeling better_! Unfortunately, once they stopped their medications, they noticed they began feeling worse! This is because their medications were playing a big role in how good they were feeling. If you believe you may not need medications anymore, ask your physician about lowering your dose. They will be able to reduce your dose in small increments to see how lowering the dose affects you. If you're still feeling good, perhaps you can keep going lower. But if you start feeling bad, you can easily return to your original dose and avoid a mental health relapse.

Consider making a pros and cons list. If you are not sure your medications are helpful for you, do not abruptly discontinue them. Instead, write a pros and cons list and discuss your results with your psychiatric provider.

Pros and Cons of Taking Medication

Pros	Cons

Avoiding Drugs and Alcohol

Recreational drugs, alcohol, and medications used more than prescribed are frequently taken to feel better. This is understandable, as drugs and alcohol work quickly and often do change our moods. However, drugs and alcohol are notorious for making mental health symptoms, including symptoms of psychosis, worse, and often create new problems (for example, legal, health, financial). We strongly advise avoiding drugs and alcohol and encourage you to reach out for help or support if you are struggling with substance use.

Here's how substance use contributed to Alan's psychosis:

I used to smoke weed every night before bed to help me fall asleep. If I had nothing going on that day, I'd smoke it in the daytime too. It usually made me feel really relaxed, but sometimes I would get really restless and on edge. Occasionally, I could hear my neighbors talking through the wall. I couldn't really make out what they were saying, but I thought maybe they knew I was smoking in the apartment and were talking about me. When I would see them in the hall, I felt uncomfortable, like something was off. When they'd make eye contact with me, I felt like they might be judging me. Eventually I began really focusing on what they might be saying or doing. I started to think they might be plotting ways to get me evicted, and that snowballed into thinking they might be trying to harm me. I spent so much time thinking about what they might be up to and how to protect myself in case they broke in. It got so bad I barely left my apartment.

Tip: If you suspect drugs or alcohol may be making your symptoms worse, but are not entirely sure, try logging what you notice before and after use. You can also check out our substance use and psychosis resources online: http://www.newharbinger.com/53394.

Managing Stress

Stress is a natural part of life. While some stress can help keep us motivated and active, chronic stress has been linked to adverse physical and mental health effects, including worsening symptoms of psychosis.

Signs your body may be stressed include:

- headaches or muscle aches

- upset stomach

- fatigue

- irritability

- increased anxiety

- trouble sleeping.

BREATHING OUT STRESS

Incorporating the healthy habits in this chapter into your daily routine is a great way to proactively manage your stress, but what if you find yourself needing some stress relief now? Taking a moment to pause and take some deep breaths when you notice symptoms of stress can help lower your heart rate and reverse your stress response (also known as the fight-or-flight response).

Practice deep breathing using the exercises below.

Star Breathing

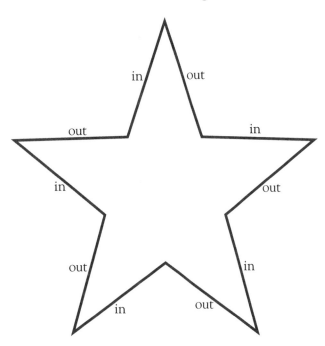

Slowly trace your finger over each line on the star as you breathe in and out.

Repeat as needed.

Square Breathing

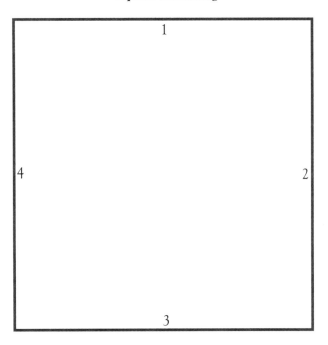

Begin by exhaling for four seconds. Pause for four seconds. Inhale for four seconds. Pause for four seconds.

Repeat as needed.

STRESS FIRST AID

Symptoms of psychosis and stress can be overwhelming. If you find yourself feeling panicked, excessively restless, or in need of some quick stress relief, try these tools for a crisis:

- **Release extra energy with exercise.** When we are very stressed, more intense exercise, like running, doing push-ups, or jumping rope, can help quickly relieve stress.

- **Cool down.** If your mind is overwhelmed, try placing an ice pack on your chest. Your mind will be automatically redirected to the cold sensation.

- **Call for help.** If you feel unsafe, including if you have strong urges to hurt yourself or someone else, call for help. For immediate help, you can call 911 or 988 (National Suicide Prevention Line). You may also call your state's local warm line (http://warmline.org). A warm line is a free service that will connect you to a mental health specialist.

Taking Care of Your Mind by Practicing Mindfulness

Mindfulness is the practice of focusing your attention (usually on the present moment) without judgment. Regularly taking time to slow down and check in with yourself through guided mindfulness exercises has been found to help reduce overall symptoms of psychosis, including lessening distress associated with voices, improving feelings of depression or anxiety, and reducing negative symptoms of psychosis (Ellett 2023). It has also been associated with reducing impulsivity and feeling more in control of your emotions (Tang et al. 2016). However, the goal of mindfulness is not to necessarily relieve distress (although this is certainly a welcomed benefit). Instead, mindfulness helps us get in touch with ourselves in a deeper way and can often help us change our relationship with any painful or uncomfortable feelings or symptoms we experience. For example, instead of working to avoid or reject these feelings, mindfulness can help us learn to accept them as part of life without getting caught up in them. It is a powerful tool and our second building block of mental wellness.

Below, we will walk you through a mindfulness exercise. Before you read on, we recommend going somewhere where you will not be interrupted for the next five to ten minutes so you can give yourself your complete attention. Start this exercise by reading through the directions. As you get more practice with this exercise, you will no longer need to read the instructions and can practice this exercise with your eyes closed.

Guided Mindfulness Exercise

Begin by taking a long exhale. Next, direct your attention to your breath. Notice how your abdomen contracts and expands as you breathe. Notice how your breath feels as it enters and exits your nose. Does it feel cool? Warm? Keep your focus on your breath. If your mind starts to wander, gently guide your focus back to your breath. You may have to do this over and over again. Keep coming back to your breath.

Focus on your breath for a couple of minutes.

Next, move your attention to your thoughts. Ask yourself, What is going through my mind right now? *Take a few moments to notice the content of your thoughts. Notice your thoughts without judging them or judging yourself for having them. How might you describe these thoughts? Are they fast? Jumbled? Loud? Are these thoughts about things that may happen (future-focused)? Things that have happened (past-focused)? Or things that are currently happening? Are you experiencing any judgmental thoughts? Notice these, too.*

Focus on your thoughts for a couple of minutes.

Now, pay attention to any feelings or emotions that arise. If it helps, use your body as a guide. For example, tension and increased heart rate may be a sign you are feeling anxious or angry. Feeling heaviness or tiredness may signal sadness. What emotions are you experiencing in this moment? Name these emotions as they come up. They are not good or bad emotions. They are simply emotions that you are experiencing right now. Notice and describe them without judging them. If your mind starts to wander away from your emotions, bring them gently back to your emotions.

Focus on your emotions for a couple of minutes.

Finally, notice any impulses you have. What do you wish to do next? Do you have an urge to do something else? What urges are you experiencing right now? Observe these urges with a sense of curiosity. You don't have to act on these urges. Just notice them.

Focus on your urges for a minute or so.

When you are ready, open your eyes and take in the space around you. Thank yourself for taking some time to check in with yourself. Note that the more you practice this exercise, the better you will get at identifying your thoughts, feelings, and urges in a mindful way. We will come back to the practice of mindfulness throughout this workbook.

Taking Care of Your Heart Through Self-Compassion

Our final building block for mental wellness is self-compassion. Self-compassion refers to being kind, supportive, and forgiving to yourself—especially when you notice you are being hard on yourself or have just experienced a setback. You can practice self-compassion by speaking to yourself in an encouraging and respectful way, by taking care of your needs as they arise, and by honoring the boundaries you set for yourself.

Adopting an attitude of self-compassion will help keep you motivated as you practice the remaining skills in this workbook and can help lessen symptoms of psychosis by reducing your overall psychological stress. For example, consider Isla's story, below:

> I was raised in a home filled with fighting. My parents often yelled at me when I made mistakes, so it's no wonder that I internalized their name-calling. I sometimes hear their voices in my head telling me that I am "no good" and "pathetic" when I feel I've done something wrong. For as long as I can remember, I've struggled with self-esteem. I'm quick to apologize and have a hard time accepting compliments. I feel like I'm constantly in a state of shame. In therapy, I'm working on being more assertive—basic stuff like making eye contact with people and walking with my shoulders back. I'm also practicing identifying when I am mean to myself and standing up to my inner critic.

It is normal to feel discouraged when you encounter a setback; however, Isla's bad feelings were made worse by her shaming inner critic. The extra stress caused by her negative self-talk contributed to increased voices. This made setbacks feel exhausting and overwhelming.

Many people struggle with a harsh inner critic that keeps them feeling discouraged. Fortunately, just like any other psychological skill, self-compassion can be improved with practice. Here are some ways Isla was able to practice self-compassion.

Be your own best friend. Isla began paying close attention to the things she said to herself and made an effort to speak to herself as if she were her own best friend. When she noticed a harsh thought, she took a moment to respond to it in a compassionate way, such as:

Original thought: *I am so stupid.*

Compassionate comeback: *It's okay to make mistakes, everyone does. I can always try again.*

Original thought: *You'll never achieve anything.*

Compassionate comeback: *I haven't reached my goal yet, but if I keep trying, I am confident I will.*

Take care of you. Isla also began prioritizing self-care, or engaging in activities that helped her feel restored and fulfilled. Self-care includes things we cover in this chapter, such as making sure you're getting enough sleep and physical activity, as well as doing things you enjoy, such as engaging in a hobby or spending time with people you like.

By making these seemingly small changes, Isla noticed that over time her inner monologue became gentler and more self-compassionate. She still felt discouraged when she encountered a setback; however, she found it much easier to get back up and try again.

Building Awareness: What are some ways you could show care for yourself in your words and actions?

_____

_____

_____

_____

_____

Summary

In this chapter, you learned about three foundational building blocks for mental wellness: healthy habits, mindfulness, and self-compassion. Each serves an important role in your overall wellness. You now have a strong foundation to begin building your own mental health toolbox, filled with coping skills for psychosis. Coping skills are things you can do to lessen the intensity of a symptom as it is occurring. The remainder of this workbook will focus on coping skills for the major symptom categories of psychosis (hallucinations, delusions, and so forth) and associated problems. We will start by focusing on the distress associated with hearing voices.

CHAPTER 4.

Coping with Voices
and Other Hallucinations

"Do you hear voices?" If you've entered the mental health system, you've probably been asked this question. Hearing voices is a relatively common human experience that we are all capable of experiencing; roughly ten to fifteen out of one hundred people experience auditory hallucinations at some point in their lives (Volpato et al. 2022). Even on antipsychotic medication, many people still hear voices, though medications can help make them more tolerable if they are distressing or distracting.

If hearing voices does not interfere with your life or bother you, then hearing voices is not a problem. You may even find it to be comforting or helpful. However, for some people, hearing voices can be incredibly painful. If you find voice-hearing to be distressing, then we believe you will benefit from the coping skills and exercises in this chapter. It is not easy to cope with hostile voices. You have already demonstrated tremendous courage and resilience!

The majority of this chapter discusses coping skills for voices, as they are the most common type of hallucination and tend to be quite upsetting for most people, although we also touch on coping with other types of hallucinations. We encourage you to practice the exercises in this chapter many times to find what works best for you and to keep practicing until the skills feel automatic. By doing so, you will be able to manage hallucinations of all types more effectively.

What Causes Voice-Hearing?

We don't know exactly what causes voice-hearing. We do know, however, that hearing voices is associated with past trauma, grief, substance use, sleep deprivation, hearing impairment, traumatic brain injury, physical illness, and mental illness (McCarthy-Jones 2012). If you experienced trauma as a child, you are more likely to hear voices (Varese et al. 2012). Research suggests a history of childhood sexual abuse can make you especially vulnerable to hearing voices (Sheffield et al. 2013). However, many people who hear voices have not experienced childhood trauma.

Biomedical and Neuropsychological Explanations

Several biomedical theories have been proposed about why people hear voices, highlighting differences in the brain's structure and functioning. For example, studies have demonstrated activation in the auditory cortex and language-related brain regions associated with hearing voices (Allen et al. 2012; Modinos et al. 2013; Planiyappan et al. 2012). Interestingly, both *Broca's area*, which is involved in inner speech production, and *Wernicke's area*, which is involved in understanding speech, have been shown to be active during voice-hearing, which is thought to support an *inner speech model* of voice hearing. According to this model, voices are your own inner speech that are (mis)perceived to be coming from outside of yourself (Frith 1992). This model doesn't explain the content of voices, or how some seem to have their own distinct personalities, however.

Psychological and Environmental Explanations

In contrast, psychological and environmental explanations focus more on the content of voices. Sigmund Freud, the founder of psychoanalysis, initially believed that hallucinations were the products of forgotten traumatic experiences from childhood. He later argued that hallucinations were reflections of fantasies. According to him, "Wishing ends with hallucinations" (Eigen 2005, 41). More broadly, psychoanalysts have viewed hallucinations as similar to dreams, capable of reflecting unresolved conflicts, fears, or desires. Additionally, the Hearing Voices Movement, a human rights movement that sees hearing voices as a normal variation of human experience, conceptualizes hearing voices as understandable in the context of a person's life (Corstens et al. 2014).

Spiritual and Other Explanations

People have been hearing voices for several millennia. Socrates, an ancient Greek philosopher, was reportedly guided by his voices, including an "oracle." Several people have pointed out that the originators of Western monotheistic religions, such as Moses, Jesus, and Mohammed, all heard voices. Until the eighteenth century, the most common explanation for voice-hearing was based on a spiritual explanation (McCarthy-Jones et al. 2013). We have also heard people speculate that they hear the voices of spirits or ghosts and loved ones who have passed away.

If you have ever wondered if you had suddenly developed the ability to hear others' thoughts due to extrasensory perception, such as clairvoyance and telepathy, then you have considered a parapsychological explanation for hearing voices.

Perhaps voice-hearing is caused by secret technology used by the government for surveillance and control. Some wonder about microchips planted in the brain, teeth, or throat. Although there is no evidence that voice-hearing is caused by such technology, this remains a compelling explanation for many in a world that has become very dependent on modern technology.

Given the lack of evidence for spiritual, parapsychological, and technological explanations, these explanations are unlikely to be supported by mental health professionals. We include them here because they are often endorsed by our clients. Regardless of your explanation, you can explore your experiences and gain insight from them.

Building Awareness: Of the explanations above, what makes the most sense to you? How do you explain the voices that you hear? How have your explanations changed over time?

_____

_____

_____

_____

_____

_____

_____

_____

Getting to Know Your Voices

Getting to know your voices—including learning when you are likely to hear them and what they are likely to say—can often make them seem more predictable. The exercises in this section will help you get to know your voices by prompting you to explore your voices more fully.

Building Awareness: When did you start hearing voices? What was going on at the time?

_____

_____

_____

_____

_____

_____

_____

How many voices do you typically hear? Describe each of their characteristics (such as gender, age, personality). Write down what you know about them.

_____

_____

_____

_____

_____

_____

_____

_____

What do your voices typically say?

_____

_____

_____

_____

_____

_____

_____

_____

How do you typically respond to your voices? (How do you feel? What do you think? What do you do?)

_____

_____

_____

_____

_____

_____

_____

_____

Use the space below to draw your voices. What do you imagine they look like?

Identifying Triggers

There are many things that can bring on or make voices worse, otherwise known as *triggers*. Check off triggers for your voices from the list below:

☐ Being in a crowd

☐ Watching TV

☐ Listening to the radio

☐ Feeling anxious

☐ Taking public transportation

☐ Going to a party

☐ Drinking coffee

☐ Using cannabis

☐ Staying in your room

☐ Meeting new people

☐ Taking medication (specify: _____)

☐ Family gatherings

☐ Talking to your counselor

☐ Being in conflict with someone

☐ Forgetting to take your medication

☐ Going on a date

☐ Using the bathroom

☐ Having sexual thoughts

☐ Other: _____

☐ Other: _____

☐ Other: _____

Now that you understand more about your voice-hearing experiences, you can start to figure out how to have more control of your experiences. For example, you can avoid your triggers or use a coping skill when you encounter a trigger. This can help you figure out how you want to respond to your voices. As you practice various coping techniques, continue to approach your experiences with curiosity and openness.

Coping with Voices and Other Hallucinations

The remainder of this chapter focuses on strategies to cope with voices and other hallucinations. Thankfully, a number of strategies have been developed by voice-hearers and mental health professionals to ease the distress associated with voice-hearing. We have grouped these strategies into the following five categories:

1. Distraction

2. Mindfulness

3. Checking it out

4. Changing your relationship with voices

5. Finding meaning in voice-hearing

Please keep in mind this is not an exhaustive list of strategies or skills. We are excited to learn more from others and add to this list over time. Some of the strategies and skills were developed for other types of problems (such as anxiety and depression) and have been shown to be effective with voice-hearing. More exercises can be found online: http://www.newharbinger.com/53394.

Distraction

Distraction is what we do when we are trying to get our mind off things that may be bothering us. We do this by *refocusing* our attention on something else. We recommend choosing activities that are enjoyable or challenging (but not so challenging that you end up feeling extremely frustrated or defeated), leading to feelings of pleasure or mastery, respectively. Sometimes wearing earplugs will decrease the volume of voices or make it easier to focus on other things. Additionally, engaging your vocal cords (by humming, reading out loud, or singing) may also help decrease the volume of voices. Distraction can also involve listening to music, talking with other people, engaging in a hobby or activity, learning a new skill, and engaging in self-care (such as relaxation techniques, showering). Distraction is a powerful tool that can be helpful for hearing voices and for other types of hallucinations as well. What are some activities that you can use to distract yourself from distressing hallucinations?

_____

_____

_____

_____

_____

_____

_____

_____

_____

Mindfulness

Mindfulness helps increase awareness, while lessening distress. Mindfulness is about taking a step back and paying attention to your voices without judgment, helping you avoid getting caught up in what your voices have to say. When you are hearing voices, follow the instructions below:

1. Start by focusing on your breath. Observe the air traveling into your nose first and then traveling further down to your chest and belly. Notice how the air is cooler going in and then warmer going out. Continue focusing on your breath for a couple of minutes.

2. Next, turn your attention to your voices:

    *   Are they loud or soft?
    *   Are the voices talking fast or slowly?
    *   What is the tone of your voices?
    *   Are they deep or high?
    *   Do they seem to be coming from inside your head or from outside of your head?

3. If thoughts or emotions start to come up for you, simply bring your attention back to noticing your voices. If you start to focus on the content of the voices or your mind starts to tell a story about them, bring your attention back to how they sound to you. Do this for at least five minutes (you can start to increase this amount over time in increments of five minutes).

4. Return to focusing on your breath. Notice how you can focus on both your breath and your voices in a similar way. When you are ready, slowly open your eyes and take in your surroundings.

Checking It Out

Checking things out can be a very powerful strategy for managing your reactions to what your voices say. When your voices tell you things that are distressing in some way, it can be helpful to ask yourself, *Is this totally true?* We can evaluate whether something is true or not by weighing the evidence. Evidence should be factual (known to be true, not just based on interpretation), objective (not influenced by personal feelings or opinions), and fairly certain (known for sure). It is important to only include solid evidence when trying to decide if something is true or not. Otherwise, you may come to a false conclusion. Take a moment to list the evidence for and against something bothersome that your voice has said in the table below.

	Evidence For	Evidence Against
What the Voices Say: _____ _____ _____		

Weigh the evidence for and against and write a statement below that accurately summarizes the evidence (as it relates to what the voice says).

_____

_____

_____

We can also use weighing the evidence to explore what we believe to be true about voices. In the following table, fill out evidence for and against the beliefs _my voices are powerful_ and _my voices are trustworthy_. We chose to focus on these two beliefs since they likely influence how you respond to your voices. We encourage you to fill this out over time as you learn more about your voices and gather more evidence (both for and against).

Evidence That Your Voices Are Powerful	Evidence That Your Voices Are Not Powerful

Weigh the evidence for and against and write a statement below that accurately summarizes how powerful you think your voices are.

_____

_____

_____

Evidence That Your Voices Are Trustworthy	Evidence That Your Voices Are Not Trustworthy

Weigh the evidence for and against and write a statement below that accurately summarizes how trustworthy you think your voices are.

_____

_____

_____

Sometimes people obey their voices because they are afraid of the consequences if they don't obey them. In the space below, write down what you think would happen if you disobeyed your voices.

_____

_____

_____

_____

_____

_____

What has happened in the past when you disobeyed your voices?

_____

_____

_____

_____

_____

If you find that you often obey your voices despite the negative consequences, we encourage you to consider testing out what happens when you do not obey them. Record your results in the space below. Disobeying commands from voices can be extremely challenging—seek additional support if needed. The more you practice disobeying your voices, the easier it will become.

_____

_____

_____

_____

_____

Changing Your Relationship with Voices

The fourth strategy includes two separate skills designed to change your relationship with voices: setting boundaries with voices and having compassion for voices. By changing your relationship with your voices, you may find that the power dynamic changes and you feel a greater sense of power or control over them. Changing your relationship with your voices is likely to be most helpful if you have a conflictual relationship with your voices and find that you spend a lot of time focusing on them.

SETTING BOUNDARIES WITH VOICES

Different styles of communication tend to lead to different results. In general, we are most likely to get what we want when we use an assertive communication style. However, it is not guaranteed that we will always get our way. Here are common styles of communication (Alberti and Emmons 2008).

Passive. This style of communication conveys the message "your needs are more important than mine." When it comes to voices, being passive with them may mean that you do what they tell you to do (even if you don't want to), or that you try to appease them (for example, by agreeing with what they have to say, even if you don't believe it).

Aggressive. This style of communication conveys the message "my needs are more important than yours." Being aggressive with voices means swearing at them, threatening to kill them, and so forth. This may also include shouting at them and even punching things—even yourself—in frustration with them. While sometimes aggressive behavior leads to getting what we want, in the long term it tends to lead to outcomes we don't (for example, loss of relationships, feelings of anger). It is not uncommon for people to be aggressive with their voices, though it may lead to increasingly more negative experiences with voices.

Passive-aggressive. Passive-aggressive communication combines aspects of passive and aggressive communication. When we use this style of communication, we may act indirectly to convey that we are upset at someone or something. For example, we might say we are not mad at someone, then completely ignore them. Similarly, it may mean promising to do what the voices say, then not doing it.

Assertive. Assertive communication conveys respect both for the other person and for yourself. It conveys the message "both of our needs are important." Assertiveness is associated with positive outcomes, such as achieving our desired outcomes and feeling good about our actions.

Building Awareness: What style of communication do you most use with the people in your life? What style of communication do you most often use with your voices?

_____

_____

_____

Being assertive with your voices means treating both your voices and you with respect. It may mean standing up for yourself and setting limits. Below are examples of what voices might say and assertive responses.

What the Voices Say	Assertive Response
"You're a loser."	"I'm not a loser. I don't believe that." "I'd rather you not say that."
"I hate you."	"I'm sorry to hear that." "That's not a nice thing to say."
"Punch him."	"No, I won't do that." "No, thank you."
"You're better than everyone else."	"Thanks, but I don't believe I am better than anyone."
"I control you."	"No, I control myself."
"You deserve to drink alcohol or use drugs."	"I would rather not. I'm determined to stay sober."
"Your daughter hates you."	"It sometimes does feel like that, but I'm working to rebuild trust." "I sometimes feel this way, but I don't believe it's true."
"Kill yourself."	"I'm not going to do that." "NO."

In the table below, come up with assertive responses to things your voices say to you. Then, practice your assertive responses with your voices. Don't be discouraged if this is difficult at first. Assertiveness, like most skills, takes practice!

What the Voices Say	Assertive Response

COMPASSION FOR VOICES

Another way to change your relationship with your voices is to approach them with compassion. Compassion can be defined as the feeling that arises when you are confronted with another's suffering and feel motivated to relieve that suffering (Dalai Lama and Tutu 2001). Rather than backing away from the other person's suffering, we acknowledge it and show caring and concern. When someone approaches us in a compassionate way, we feel understood. We may also feel comforted and less alone. When faced with painful criticism, whether from others or from our voices, showing ourselves compassion can be especially powerful.

Sometimes it is difficult to come up with compassionate responses in the moment. In these situations, it can be helpful to ask, "What would _____ say?" (someone you find to be very compassionate). Alternatively, it can be helpful to think about what you might say to someone you have love and compassion for if they were in the same situation.

When you approach voices (and yourself) with compassion, you recognize that they come from a place of suffering, perhaps from someplace within you. Here is one example of approaching voices compassionately.

Voice: You're a loser. You're crazy.

Me: You frequently tell me that. It must be very important to you that I hear this.

Voice: You're nothing but a crazy loser.

Me: I hear you saying that I'm a "crazy loser." That's a painful thing for me to hear.

Voice: It's true. No one will ever want to be with you.

Me: It's very important for me to find a relationship. You've really hit on a big fear of mine.

Voice: You will die alone.

Me: Yes, that's one of my biggest fears. Do you have this fear as well?

Voice: Shut up. You sound pathetic.

Me: You sound really angry and perhaps a little scared.

Voice: I'm not scared. Don't try to turn this around on me.

Me: It's okay. I can relate to feeling angry and scared. I have felt this a lot.

Voice: Shut up, loser. You're pathetic.

Me: You're coming from a place of suffering. I recognize that now.

Finding Meaning in Voice-Hearing

The last strategy is perhaps the most helpful after you have practiced the other strategies. It involves thinking of voices and what they say in a different way (similar to changing beliefs about voices). However, rather than restructuring thoughts or changing beliefs, you seek out the "hidden meaning" behind the messages. Consider Jeff's insight:

Whenever I am mad at someone, my voices tell me to kill that person. This used to be really distressing because I was afraid that I would listen to my voices and end up hurting someone. I was afraid that hearing voices made me dangerous. I realized that my voices were expressing my anger for me, and I made a commitment never to obey them. Now, whenever my voices tell me to kill someone, I acknowledge that I am upset with the other person, and I try to figure out what to do about it. Do I talk to the person about being angry with them or hurt by them? Do I try to get over it? I also know that if I can work on feeling less angry, my voices will seem less angry as well.

This strategy involves searching for the metaphorical meaning behind what the voices say instead of the literal meaning. When we take something literally, we do not search for the meaning behind it. So, if we hear a voice say, "I'm going to kill your family," we believe that there is someone or something that wants to kill our family. Naturally, we become scared or angry. But what if we were to take this metaphorically, or as representing something else? Here are some possibilities for what this message might represent:

- Fear that you have about the safety of your loved ones (in a dangerous world)

- Fear that you have about changing relationships that you have with your loved ones (ending of our current, existing relationships)

- Unexpressed anger that you have for your family members (not that you literally want to harm them—you're just upset with them)

What about when voices say, "Kill yourself!"? What are some possible ways to interpret this message? Possible interpretations include:

- I am suffering a lot right now.

- There are things that I need to change in my life.

- I am really angry at myself.

- This reflects feelings of shame associated with my past or my mental illness.

The next time you hear voices, ask yourself, *What could be the meaning behind this?* Further questions include:

- *Could this represent a fear that I have?*

- *Could this represent a wish that I have?*

- *Could this represent a belief that I have?*

- *Is this related to something I experienced in my past?*

- *What purpose does this message serve?*

This is a very different reaction from taking voices at face value and believing what they say. Use the table below to try out this skill. Try to come up with two possible meanings for each phrase you are focusing on.

What the Voices Say	Possible Meaning Behind This

Coping with Other Hallucinations

Although the majority of this chapter focused on coping with voices, we acknowledge that other types of hallucinations can be just as upsetting. For example, seeing disturbing images or feeling like someone or something is poking at your skin can be particularly unsettling. The skills we've covered here can be applied to other types of hallucinations, for example, engaging in distraction and offering yourself reassurance when you notice a tactile hallucination. In particular, we want to highlight how mindfulness can be used to cope with other types of hallucinations.

The next time you experience a hallucination, focus on the details and describe the hallucination as much as possible, without judgment. For example, if you see an image in front of you, describe the image out loud using descriptive terms. Or better yet, write down what you are seeing, including the shapes and colors of the image. Describe the image in vivid detail so that someone who is not able to see the image can imagine exactly what you are seeing. Can you approach the image with interest? If you notice intense thoughts and feelings coming up in response to the image or sensation, can you describe these as well, again, without judgment? Putting some distance between yourself and these experiences can also make them more manageable. For example, rather than stating, "I see a spider!", you can state, "I am having the experience of seeing a spider," or "I'm experiencing a visual hallucination in the form of a spider."

Does the image or sensation remind you of other images and sensations from your past? If so, it may be helpful to explore these associations, perhaps with a therapist, peer specialist, or friend. Finding meaning in the experience may help you understand the experience better and why it may be recurring.

Summary

In this chapter, we covered the important topic of coping with voices. We encouraged you to get to know your voices and explore your beliefs about them. The goal is not to get rid of voices, but to learn how to cope with them better. These skills take practice, so please be patient with yourself as you practice them (we have included blank templates for the exercises in this chapter on the website for this book: http://www.newharbinger.com/53394). Find what works best for you. Remember that you are not alone. Many of these strategies and skills have been developed by others who have struggled with their voices. Over time, you may find these experiences less distressing and perhaps personally meaningful. Next, we introduce coping skills for delusional thoughts and beliefs.

CHAPTER 5

Coping with Paranoid and Other "Delusional" Beliefs

In chapter 1, we noted that psychosis results in a loss of touch with reality, or a state of mind in which it is hard to differentiate between what is real and not real, or false. This occurs in part because psychosis changes *how* your mind works and subsequently *what* you think and believe.

In this chapter, we explore how psychosis impacts your thinking and offer interventions to help you better distinguish between objective reality (based on evidence and usually shared by others) and what may be a false belief, or a delusion. Unlike a thought, which can be considered a transitory piece of information that goes through our minds—one that we may or may not pay attention to or react to—a delusion refers to a belief. Beliefs represent things we feel to be true or feel very strongly about.

Because delusional beliefs can continue to feel completely true even when they lack solid evidence, or have evidence that contradicts them, it is often difficult to get rid of them completely. Therefore, we offer interventions to help you better manage the incredible impact these beliefs can have on your life, including how to:

- Spend less of your time and energy on these beliefs to regain a sense of balance

- Learn ways to cope with the distress these beliefs can cause

- Explore the potential meaning and function behind your beliefs.

Even if you don't have a delusion, we encourage you to continue reading because the exercises in this chapter can be applied to any thought or belief that could be considered time-consuming, emotionally draining, or unhelpful. Tuning into your thoughts and actively challenging them takes practice, patience, and courage, but the payoff is well worth the investment. Return to this chapter anytime you need support coping with distressing thoughts or beliefs.

The How: Psychosis's Impact on Your Perception

How exactly psychosis changes the brain is yet to be completely understood. However, researchers have consistently observed multiple changes to the neurotransmitter dopamine during psychosis. One of dopamine's many roles is to help you determine what is *salient*, or important to focus on—this includes telling you what external things to pay attention to as well as alerting you to potentially important internal experiences, such as memories, feelings, and sensations (Winton-Brown et al. 2014).

This means that when you experience psychosis, you will notice changes to what catches your attention or what feels directed at you. Indeed, one of the earliest signs of psychosis is feeling like something is off, something is not right, or something strange is going on. You may feel like you are at the center of something, but cannot figure out what, which can be disturbing, confusing, and stressful. It makes good sense that in this state, your mind would be working overtime to explain what is happening!

However, the conclusions reached during an episode of psychosis are often incorrect because they have been heavily influenced by the dysregulated dopamine system (a state of hyper-salience). This combined with other symptoms of psychosis, such as hallucinations, can lead you to draw false conclusions about what is going on or explanations that make sense to you, but ones that the people around you are unlikely to agree with. This can leave you feeling isolated and frustrated while your support system struggles to know how best to help.

See Shannon's story, below, describing how encountering an ambiguous situation (vague neck pain) in a state of hyper-salience contributed to the development of a false conclusion. We put a star (*) next to examples of how Shannon was paying special attention to something she likely would not have if she were not in a hyper-salient state:

About a year before my diagnosis, I started noticing a pain in my neck. The pain would come on suddenly and last a few seconds before disappearing. It made me anxious because I didn't know if it was something serious or not. One day my friend came over, and I noticed that the pain in my neck flared up any time she was showing me something on her phone.* At one point, she looked at me and smiled,* as if she knew something I didn't. Later I noticed the same thing happened when my husband showed me his phone.* I started thinking that a device had been implanted in my neck and that other people were able to activate it with their cell phone. Everywhere I looked, there seemed to be evidence that supported my belief—people looking at me strangely in stores*; people saying, "What a pain in the neck"*; things like that. Whenever my husband would touch his neck,* I thought he might be trying to tell me covertly about the device. I figured he must have felt guilty for what he had done. Eventually I cut into my neck to try to remove the device, which is what ended up prompting my family to get me help.

Shannon wished to better understand the source of her neck pain. She paid more attention to her pain when cell phones were present. If she were not in a state of hyper-salience, Shannon would have likely explained the relationship between her neck pain and viewing a cell phone as *I need to bend my neck to look down at the phone, which aggravates the pain.* However, because psychosis creates a hyper-salient state that makes everyday things feel much more significant and personal, she instead made sense of the correlation by telling herself that a device had been implanted in her neck. This belief understandably caused her significant distress and eventually led to her hurting herself.

Building Awareness: Can you identify times when you focused on something in your environment that perhaps wasn't as significant as you thought? What were you focusing on? What were the consequences of this?

_____

_____

_____

_____

_____

_____

_____

_____

_____

The What: Types of Thoughts That May Occur with Psychosis

Your mental state impacts the content of your thoughts. For example, when you are depressed, your thoughts will often reflect themes of sadness, hopelessness, or guilt. When you're anxious, your thoughts will alert you to things that could go wrong. During an episode of psychosis, your thoughts will generally fit into one of the following themes: grandiose, religious, paranoid, referential, and control (Bentall 2024).

Research has shown that these themes appear to be universal for people experiencing psychosis, meaning they occur across cultures (Bentall 2024). Bentall writes, "One possible interpretation of this finding is that the themes reflect common existential themes that affect all humankind, such as the need to distinguish between trustworthy and untrustworthy others (paranoia), the need to make sense of ambiguous communications (reference), and concerns about social rank and the meaning of life (grandiose and religious)" (9).

Below are examples of common grandiose, religious, paranoid, referential, and control beliefs that occur with psychosis. As you read the lists, you may notice that some beliefs could fit in more than one category. For example, the belief *other people can read my thoughts* (referential) could very well cause feelings of paranoia. What is most important here is learning to recognize the major categories of common thoughts and beliefs that occur with psychosis so you can more quickly identify when they are occurring. Then, you can prompt yourself to use one or more of the coping skills covered later in this chapter.

Read the lists below and check off any beliefs you have noticed in your own thinking.

Grandiose

Grandiose beliefs have to do with power, status, and influence. They are generally exciting to experience and can boost your mood and self-esteem.

☐ *I am a celebrity or famous person* (such as a musician, politician, or movie star).

☐ *I have a powerful role* (for example, *I am an FBI or CIA agent, I am a CEO of a major company*).

☐ *I am very rich.*

☐ *Someone I admire is in love with me* (this can include the belief that you are in a relationship with a famous person).

☐ *I have a powerful talent* (for example, *I can heal others, I can control the weather, I am responsible for saving the world or others*).

☐ *I have made an important discovery* (for example, invented a cure for a disease, solved a major social problem, exposed a major scandal).

Religious or Spiritual

Religious beliefs may relate to any of the major religions or other spiritual practices and metaphysical possibilities. They may engender a range of emotions, from feeling at peace or feeling powerful, to feeling overwhelmed and distressed.

☐ *I am God. I am a god.*

☐ *I am the devil. I am a demon.*

☐ *I am a powerful spiritual entity or figure* (such as an angel, disciple, or prophet).

☐ *God is using me for a special purpose.*

☐ *I am featured in the Bible, Quran, or another holy text.*

☐ *Others have supernatural powers or are associated with the devil or an evil entity* (this can also include the belief that you have been cursed, possessed, or are being controlled by magic).

☐ *We are living in a metaverse or parallel universe.*

Paranoid

Paranoid beliefs relate to your safety, including your physical safety, emotional safety, and financial safety. These beliefs are the most common type of delusion (Bentall 2024) and can be extremely disturbing and upsetting to experience.

☐ *People are tracking me or surveilling me* (includes the belief you are being gang-stalked or that drones are monitoring you).

☐ *Something has been implanted in me* (for example, a microchip, tracking device, objects, or another person).

☐ *My partner is cheating on me.*

☐ *People are stealing, touching, or moving my belongings behind my back.*

☐ *Someone is stealing my organs or my body parts.*

☐ *Other people are imposters of close friends, family, or acquaintances* (also known as Capgras syndrome).

☐ *Someone or something is sexually violating me in my sleep.*

☐ *People don't mean what they say, are talking about me, or are making passive aggressive threats or insults toward me.*

☐ *People are trying to harm me or want me dead.*

☐ *My food or environment has been poisoned or contaminated.*

☐ *The people around me are actually actors working to deceive me.*

Referential

Referential beliefs involve interpreting things in your environment as having a special meaning for you.

☐ *The people in my environment and I are part of a shared mind: we have the same thoughts.*

☐ *People can read my thoughts.*

☐ *Strangers are paying special attention to me.*

☐ *The television, radio, or other electronic device is watching me or communicating with me.*

☐ *People on the television can see me and are reacting to me.*

Control

Control beliefs cause you to feel as if you have lost control of some part of yourself or your entire self. These beliefs are thought to be closely related to hallucinations because your inner experiences are being attributed to something outside of yourself (Bentall 2024).

☐ *Someone or something (for example, another person, a force, a device, or an entity) is controlling my behavior, mood, or energy.*

☐ *Someone or something is putting thoughts into my head or taking thoughts out.*

☐ *I have no free will. I am a device that is being used.*

Is This Thought Influenced by Your Psychosis?

Now that you have a better sense of how psychosis can influence your thinking, the skills in this section will help you slow down and examine your thoughts more closely. Taking time to explore your thoughts can help you (1) avoid jumping to conclusions, (2) develop multiple possibilities for what may be happening, and (3) figure out if your thoughts are true or not.

Avoid Jumping to Conclusions by Checking Your Thought

Our brains are excellent at making quick judgment calls. This ability helps us avoid getting bogged down by overanalyzing each and every situation we encounter. In many situations, this efficient approach is unlikely to cause us any problems. However, if we jump to a conclusion that is false, we can find ourselves unnecessarily distressed or, in extreme cases, acting on these beliefs and suffering the consequences.

Notice how Mil's thought and subsequent behavior cost him his freedom:

I was driving home from work and saw a license plate that had three 6's on it. My first thought was, The driver is the devil and is trying to provoke me. I can't let this continue. I followed him for about ten miles before confronting him in his driveway. I yelled at him, and we started fighting. I ended up in jail, where I was found incompetent to stand trial. I spent almost a year in the state hospital learning legal skills. I was never a confrontational person before, but I just got so swept away by my anger.

In the following table, identify a troubling thought or belief that you would like to "check out." Then answer the following questions. A copy of this worksheet is also included on the website for this book, http://www.newharbinger.com/53394, so you can use it more than once.

Thought to be explored:	
Question to Ask Yourself	**Your Reply**
What facts do I have to support this thought being true?	
What facts do I have to support this thought being false?	
Am I making any assumptions? If so, what are they?	
Is this thought based mostly on feelings? (For example, "I felt lonely and noticed the thought, *I will never find a relationship*.") If so, what feelings?	
How might other people interpret this situation?	

What other possibilities are there?	
Could this be an exaggeration or worst-case scenario? If so, what is the most likely scenario?	
Do you feel you need more information to support or disprove your thought? If so, what information would be helpful?	

Developing Alternative Explanations

Putting too much weight into a single explanation can contribute to the development of a delusion. In this section, you will practice coming up with multiple explanations for ambiguous, or unclear, events.

Read the hypothetical scenarios below and list five potential explanations for what might be going on. Then, use the template to practice developing alternative explanations for ambiguous events that you have observed (and may have drawn false conclusions from).

Scenario #1. Someone you don't know approaches you in the street and tells you, "You've been chosen," then walks away. What are five explanations for this?

1. _____

2. _____

3. _____

4. _____

5. _____

Scenario #2. You are watching TV when one of the actors says your name. What are five explanations for this?

1. _____
2. _____
3. _____
4. _____
5. _____

Your scenario: _____

Your first thought: _____

Alternative explanations:

1. _____
2. _____
3. _____
4. _____
5. _____

Developing an Experiment to Test Your Thought

Behavioral experiments are another way to check out your thoughts. One reason this tool is so powerful is that it is experiential. Rather than simply weighing the evidence for and against, you are collecting evidence and testing things out. This skill is very helpful when you are unsure whether something is true or not, or if you *feel sure* something is true, but have many people in your life telling you it may be part of your psychosis.

Here's how to perform behavioral experiments:

1. **State your hypothesis.** What is the thought or belief to be tested? (This could also be something that your voices tell you if you hear voices). Make sure that the statement you are testing is something that can be verified (proven true or false).

2. **Design your experiment.** How will you verify whether this is more likely to be true or false? What steps do you need to include?

3. **Carry out your experiment.** Make sure the experiment is feasible and time-limited!

4. **Evaluate the results of your experiment.** What did you find out? Does it support your hypothesis?

5. **Identify next steps** (for example, follow-up experiments), if needed. Do you need to conduct further experiments?

Below, Cyn tested her belief that she can read other people's minds with her friend Paige:

1. **Hypothesis:** I can read other people's minds.

2. **Method:** Ask my friend, Paige, to write down a number between 1 and 100 on a piece of paper and then repeat that number in her head for fifteen seconds. Then I will guess what number she is thinking of. She will show me the number that she was thinking about.

3. **Results:** I guessed 10, and Paige had written down 42.

4. **Conclusion:** I was not able to guess what number she had been thinking of.

5. **Follow-up experiment:** I will try this again with someone else (it may be that I am only able to do this with close loved ones).

Other experiments we have tried with the people we work with include testing to see if they were really being followed or surveilled, if they were being poisoned, and seeing if something had been implanted in their skin (medical tests revealed there was nothing detectable under their skin).

Now design your own behavioral experiment to test. Note that a hypothesis can also include thoughts or predictions about yourself (for example, *I have supernatural powers*, or *Everyone is against me*).

1. **Hypothesis:** _____

    _____

2. **Method:** _____

    _____

    _____

    _____

3. Results: _____

    _____

4. Conclusion: _____

    _____

5. Follow-up experiment: _____

    _____

    _____

Getting Distance from Time-Consuming Beliefs

Delusions tend to be highly time-consuming because they provoke strong emotions, can be threatening, or may be very interesting and compelling. Becoming preoccupied, or spending a lot of time on something, can take you away from the activities and people you enjoy. Regaining a sense of balance in your life by reducing preoccupation with a delusion is an important component of recovery.

Read Jill's story to see how she became preoccupied with her belief that someone was in her home:

> In the last six months, I started feeling more anxious at home and began to get the feeling someone was sneaking in behind my back. I set up cameras to catch the person, but they always avoided detection. I'd leave work early or sometimes just call out of work altogether in hopes of catching them in the act. I didn't feel safe sleeping in my home and spent a lot of money and time at a nearby hotel. I explained my situation to my friends, family, and even the police, but they've all told me no one was breaking in. I feel totally alone with this problem and am completely overwhelmed by it.

In Jill's example, she does not have any firm evidence that someone is breaking in. However, she has a strong *feeling* that something bad is happening. This represents a threat to her safety and is understandably disturbing her sense of peace. She has become preoccupied by her belief by (1) spending a lot of time worrying about it, (2) setting up and monitoring cameras, (3) leaving work, (4) spending time and money at hotels, and (5) discussing her belief with loved ones and police. By spending so much time on this belief despite the lack of evidence to support it being true, Jill is keeping herself in a state of fear and stress when she does not need to be.

Building Awareness:

1. Is there a belief that takes up a lot of your time? If so, write it here:

    _____

    _____

2. Next, how much time would you estimate you spend on this belief per day (for example, 50 percent of your day, at least once an hour)?

    _____

3. How do you imagine your life would be different if you spent less time on this belief? Are there some things you would like to give more of your attention to going forward?

    _____

    _____

    _____

    _____

    _____

    _____

Setting Limits with Your Belief

If after completing the activity above, you've identified a thought or belief that is taking up more of your time and peace than you would like, we invite you to brainstorm ways in which you could set limits with your belief. For example, only choosing to engage with the belief during a certain time frame (for example, from 10:00 to 10:30 a.m.), choosing to ignore the belief or use a coping skill when you notice it, or choosing to reduce the amount of time you spend discussing or researching the belief.

Ways you can set limits with your belief:

_____

_____

_____

_____

_____

_____

_____

_____

Coping with Distressing Thoughts and Beliefs

Some thoughts—especially suspicious thoughts—can be incredibly overwhelming and terrifying. In this section, we review ways to get relief from thoughts that feel overwhelming or terrifying, thoughts that make you feel badly about yourself or others, or any thought that takes you away from living your life in the present moment.

Lessening the Impact of Thoughts Through Defusion

Defusion is a process of distancing ourselves from our thoughts, emotions, and sensations so we do not become "hooked," or caught up by them. It is about noticing thoughts without judgment and letting them come and go (Hayes et al. 2012). Perhaps you notice a thought that is particularly upsetting or annoying. Every time you notice this thought, you find yourself becoming stressed, imagining a cascade of worst-case scenarios. The thought has "hooked" you in that instance, like a fish that has been caught by the same bait yet again!

Defusion involves either getting "unhooked" or not biting the bait in the first place. Defusion is a technique that falls under the umbrella of mindfulness. If you notice a thought that says, *They're going to harm you*, state to yourself, *I'm having the thought that they're going to harm me*, or *I notice my mind is telling me there's a possibility they could harm me*. This will put some distance between yourself and the content of your thoughts so you are less reactive to them.

Here are some other exercises that involve defusing from thoughts. Choose a couple to practice. Notice how your experience of your thoughts changes as you put some distance between yourself (the person observing) and your thoughts.

- **Leaves on a stream.** Every time you notice a distressing thought, take it and place it onto an imaginary leaf that is floating down a stream. Continue placing such thoughts on various leaves floating down the stream and watch (in your mind's eye) as they flow down the stream.

- **Different voices.** Repeat what your thoughts have to say but say it with a different voice (for example, very deep, very high, very fast, very slow, in the voice of your favorite cartoon character). You are not trying to change the message. You are trying to change your experience of the message. Don't worry if the message is true or not. Just notice that it is a message that can be said in a lot of different ways and with a lot of different voices. You may even want to sing the message in the tune of a familiar song!

- **Thank your brain.** Say, "Thank you brain for giving me this message!" every time you notice an especially provocative thought that is difficult for you to ignore. Notice what the thought says and then, let it go.

Tip: The activities above can also be used to help you get relief from distressing voices!

Grounding and Offering Yourself Reassurance

"Grounding" refers to directing your attention to the present moment. Grounding can help us orient to reality, move away from racing or disturbing thoughts, and soothe anxious or overwhelmed feelings.

To practice grounding, start by taking some long, deep breaths. Next, take a moment to refocus your attention on each of your senses, noticing everything you see, one at a time.

First, describe what you see—colors, shapes, objects, light. What do you notice?

_____

_____

_____

_____

_____

_____

Next, tune in to what you can feel, or touch. Explore the texture, temperature, or weight. Describe it here:

_____

_____

_____

_____

_____

_____

Now, take a moment to really listen to the things around you. Are these sounds loud or soft? Close or far? Describe what you hear below:

_____

_____

_____

_____

_____

_____

What about your sense of smell? Do you notice any scents in your environment? Note these below:

_____

_____

_____

Finally, are you able to taste anything right now? Perhaps you have a favorite snack, gum, or mint nearby that you can taste. Describe any tastes you experience here:

_____

_____

_____

_____

_____

As you are grounding yourself, try repeating the sentence. "I am safe, this thought is not a fact, I am okay." Or, come up with your own grounding statement that helps keep you connected to the present moment. What are some statements that you can use to ground yourself?

_____

_____

_____

_____

_____

_____

_____

_____

_____

_____

_____

Exploring a Deeper Meaning

Finally, sometimes our thoughts reflect something deeper going on inside of us. Perhaps your belief is trying to alert you to something. Or perhaps it is trying to protect you from an unpleasant experience or emotion. What is the function of your belief? Could it be connected to something from your past that still needs to be processed? Below are examples of delusional beliefs and questions that you can ask yourself to explore what may be behind these beliefs. We have included additional questions online: http://www.newharbin ger.com/53394.

Belief	Questions to Ask Yourself
I am not myself. I have switched places with someone.	Did something happen recently that made you feel bad about yourself? Did you notice a thought, feeling, or physical sensation that was different from what you usually notice? Are you worried someone might be upset with you?
I am a famous celebrity or powerful person.	Does this person do something you would like to do? (For example, if you believe you are a famous musician, do you have an interest in music?) Were you feeling badly about yourself before you noticed this thought? Does this thought help you feel better? Did you have a dream for your future that you were not able to achieve for some reason?

Belief	Questions to Ask Yourself
Other people are out to get me.	Do you often feel different from other people or are worried you don't fit in?
	Have you been bullied or mistreated in the past?
	Do you struggle with social anxiety? If so, could this thought be a symptom of that?

What is a belief you have that is considered to be "delusional" or not true by others?

_____

_____

Brainstorm what might be behind this belief. How is it related to your previous experiences? What function does this belief serve in your life?

_____

_____

_____

_____

_____

_____

_____

If, after completing the exercise above, you feel your belief may reflect something deeper going on for you, take a moment to consider the ways you could begin addressing the underlying concern. For example:

"Delusional" belief: *I am a messenger for God and have great power.*

Underlying concern: *I have had periods in my life where I have felt powerless. I am worried I haven't lived up to my full potential.*

Ways to address the underlying concern: *I can work on building mastery by starting a project that is important to me; I can build up my self-esteem and confidence through self-care and affirmations.*

"Delusional" belief: _____

Underlying concern: _____

Ways to address the underlying concern: _____

_____

_____

_____

_____

"Delusional" belief: _____

Underlying concern: _____

Ways to address the underlying concern: _____

_____

_____

_____

_____

"Delusional" belief: _____

Underlying concern: _____

Ways to address the underlying concern: _____

_____

_____

_____

_____

Summary

In this chapter, we reviewed how psychosis contributes to the development of delusions and identified ways to work more effectively with delusional beliefs so they are less disruptive to your life. You can examine the evidence for and against your thoughts and beliefs. You can also create some distance between yourself and your thoughts and beliefs and explore the meaning behind them. Practicing these skills takes time, energy, and commitment. It can be helpful to think of recovery as a long-term process of self-exploration and self-kindness. In chapter 6, we focus on how to overcome the cognitive symptoms associated with psychosis.

Overcoming Cognitive Difficulties to Improve Your Thinking

Cognition refers to your "thinking skills"—these are the various abilities (thanks to your brain!) that allow you to learn and interact with the world around you. You use your cognitive abilities to fill out job applications and learn the tasks associated with your job. Your cognitive abilities help you figure out who you would like to get to know better (and who you allow to get to know you). Everything you do involves cognition—and psychosis can impact cognition in numerous ways. Consider Ty's story:

> I did well in school and had a lot of friends growing up. In the ninth grade, however, I started to lose my focus. My parents and teachers wondered if I was depressed—I probably was. I had a psychotic episode in my junior year of high school, and I ended up dropping out. I was treated with an antipsychotic medication and eventually received my GED. I wanted to go to college but didn't think I could focus on my schoolwork. My parents complained that I was frequently "zoning out" and "unmotivated." I sometimes left things burning on the stove and had trouble finding things... I felt really frustrated and discouraged, and I spent a lot of time in my room smoking cannabis and playing video games.

Psychosis is known to impact a variety of cognitive abilities (Bowie and Harvey 2006; Mancuso et al. 2011; Sheffield et al. 2018), including:

- **Perception**—recognizing and interpreting sensory information

- **Attention**—focusing on a task while ignoring distractions

- **Memory**—storing and retrieving information from your mind

- **Motor skills**—using your body to carry out tasks

- **Language**—understanding and producing words and sentences

- **Visual and spatial processing**—making sense of what you see, visualizing scenarios in your mind

- **Executive functioning**—engaging in goal-oriented behavior, such as decision making, planning, and problem solving

- **Processing speed**—the speed at which you process and respond to information

- **Social cognition**—the ability to understand social situations and other people.

The cognitive abilities above work together in important ways to help you complete everyday tasks. Memory, for example, requires storing information so it can be retrieved later—this requires paying attention. Sometimes, you might blame your "bad memory" on forgetting people's names, when really, it has more to do with difficulties with paying attention, especially for a prolonged period (in other words, concentrating). Learning how to drive a car requires concentration, memory, visual and spatial processing, motor skills, and executive functioning.

In this chapter, we go over ways to improve your cognitive skills. If you can relate to feeling frustrated by your cognitive abilities, then practicing the skills in this chapter will be an important part of helping you reach your recovery goals. Just as you work out physically to become stronger, have more endurance, and increase your flexibility, you can also work out your brain to improve your cognitive functioning. The first step is to identify the ways you are struggling.

Identify Your Cognitive Difficulties and Their Impact on You

Even when symptoms of psychosis are well-treated, cognitive difficulties may persist. These abilities are also impacted by stress, anxiety, lack of sleep, poor nutrition, and a sedentary lifestyle (Huang et al. 2020; Mamalaki et al. 2022). Cognitive difficulties—even more than symptoms of psychosis—are associated with difficulties functioning, including performing well in school and work, living independently, and maintaining relationships (Bowie and Harvey 2006). While some medications may be beneficial for improving cognitive difficulties, such as medications for attention deficit disorder (ADD) or attention deficit hyperactivity disorder (ADHD), you may find that you continue to experience these problems even on medications or because of them (antipsychotic medications often have side effects, such as sedation or feeling slowed down).

Below are common cognitive difficulties associated with psychosis. Make a checkmark next to any you experience.

Attention:

☐ Easily distracted

☐ Difficulty learning new things

☐ Can't concentrate on reading

☐ Trouble repeating back information you just heard (such as phone numbers)

☐ Making careless mistakes

☐ Trouble completing tasks

☐ Difficulty following directions

Memory:

☐ Difficulty remembering to take medication

☐ Misplacing things

☐ Forgetting appointments

☐ Forgetting important dates

☐ Difficulty recalling what you had for breakfast

☐ Forgetting people's names

☐ Not remembering what you read

☐ Not remembering what you watched (such as the plot of a movie)

Processing speed:

☐ Feeling like your mind is slowed down

☐ Taking more time than most people to finish tasks

☐ Trouble keeping up with conversation

☐ Taking time to answer questions

Executive functioning:

☐ Poor impulse control

☐ Difficulty with organization

☐ Poor time management

☐ Trouble making decisions

Social cognition:

☐ Trouble knowing how to act in social situations

☐ Misreading other people's facial expressions or body language

☐ Difficulty seeing other people's points of view

☐ Difficulty predicting the behavior of other people

Give Your Brain a Workout

Like working out, the more you practice cognitive exercises, the more "fit" your brain will become. Cognitive training is like weight training—there are many programs and apps designed to provide regular workouts for your brain. Cognitive training typically involves multiple training exercises (thirty to sixty minutes per session) every week for several weeks or months and is an important component of cognitive remediation therapy (CRT), a treatment that has been shown to be effective in improving the cognitive difficulties associated with mental illness, traumatic brain injuries, and aging (Cicerone et al. 2019; Sharma et al. 2016; Wykes and Spaulding 2011). Typically administered over the computer or tablet, these programs include numerous exercises to "flex" your cognitive skills and build your brain's ability to learn, manipulate, and remember information. Some of these programs are:

- CogniFit

- BrainHQ

- COGPACK

- HAPPYNeuron

You can use the programs above to work out your brain for a small monthly fee. Otherwise, you can download free apps that include cognitive exercises or make time in your day to focus your attention for sustained periods (for example, fifteen or thirty minutes). Remember, the more you practice, the easier these exercises will become, and the more improvement you are likely to see in your ability to learn and retain information, think in a more organized and clear way, and problem solve effectively. We have also seen the people we work with benefit from daily practice of activities such as sudoku, word searches, crossword puzzles, puzzles, and video games. Reading books, magazines, and newspaper articles; engaging in physical exercise; and participating in social activities can also help improve your mental fitness (Sánchez-Izquierdo and Fernández-Ballesteros 2021).

Now that you have identified which cognitive abilities you struggle with, let's identify some days and times when you could commit to working on them. What activities would you be open to trying? When could you engage in these activities?

_____

_____

_____

_____

In addition to cognitive training, CRT often includes learning strategies to improve cognitive functioning. The rest of this chapter focuses on such strategies.

Self-Management Strategies

Self-management strategies, such as staying organized, are strategies to help to make your life easier. These strategies help improve your cognition by decreasing your cognitive load and stress level. Below are some organizational strategies that may help you feel more in control of your life.

Designating a "Landing Spot"

Do you often feel disorganized? Perhaps you are running late for an appointment and feel stressed-out because you can't find your phone. Instead of asking yourself, *Why am I so disorganized?!*, create a "landing spot" near the door of your residence for the items you use frequently. This could be a bowl on a small table or a hanging basket. Get in the habit of placing the items you need daily (such as your keys, wallet, and phone) in the same spot. Where could you create a landing spot to use?

_____

_____

Routines Are Rad

Your brain loves to make connections between things! Once you enjoy the full benefit of having daily routines, hopefully you will start to associate routines with "radness" (we are using alliteration here, or the repetition of sounds at the beginning of words close together, which is one way to boost memory). A structured routine helps you organize your life and know what to expect. Structure also tends to lead to better habits, such as getting adequate sleep and exercise.

What activity would you like to make a daily habit? When is the best time to engage in this activity? Can you pair this activity with another activity that you do daily (such as pairing brushing your teeth with fifteen minutes of cognitive training)?

_____

_____

_____

_____

Write down your morning and evening routines, including any additions you would like to make to your routines.

Morning Routine

Time	Activity

Evening Routine

Time	Activity

Are there any activities you would like to make a weekly habit, such as working out at the gym, doing chores (for example, laundry once a week), or social activities (such as calling a friend or family member)? Enter all your regular weekly activities in a calendar, including all appointments, with the times you do them. If you are working toward a goal, such as finding a job, find regular times to work on it (for example, looking online for job openings or editing your resume) and include those tasks in your schedule. If you have trouble sticking to your schedule, create a new schedule that is more realistic. For example, rather than scheduling yoga four times a week if you are currently not doing yoga at all, start by scheduling yoga once a week, and build from there!

You can download a weekly schedule and print out other templates on the website for this book: http://www.newharbinger.com/53394. While there, make sure to also check out our tips on creating a personal planner, which is crucial to staying organized.

Improving Attention

Difficulty paying attention is probably the number one cognitive complaint of people who experience psychosis. This is unfortunate because attention problems can get in the way of enjoyable activities, such as reading or watching movies. The good news is that there are many ways to improve your ability to pay attention. Review the strategies below and checkmark any you are interested in trying:

- ☐ **Eliminate distractions.** When possible, eliminate potential distractions. If you are working on your computer, you can turn off email notifications or disconnect your computer from the internet.

- ☐ **Do one thing at a time.** Multitasking will slow you down and make you lose focus!

- ☐ **Take breaks.** If you are having a lot of trouble focusing, take a short break. You can stretch, take a walk, enjoy a snack, and then revisit your task. You may want to schedule breaks into a task. For example, if you are working on an assignment, spend twenty minutes on the assignment before taking a ten-minute break; then repeat. Build your stamina like you would with weight training.

- ☐ **Change your environment.** Some environments have too many distractions in them! Can't concentrate no matter how many breaks you take? Maybe it's time to change your environment—go to the library or a coffee shop, somewhere you aren't likely to be interrupted.

Mindfulness

Practicing mindfulness is another wonderful way to improve your attention (Posner et al. 2015). You can practice mindfulness anywhere: standing in line at the grocery store, walking to the bus stop, listening to music late at night with your lights turned off. Spend five minutes focusing on whatever activity you are engaged in, noticing the sensations on your skin; what you see, hear, and smell; and any thoughts or feelings that come up. Remember that mindfulness involves paying attention without judgment, so if judgment comes up, just notice it and bring your attention back to your task. Washing dishes is a common activity to practice doing mindfully. If there is a task you engage in daily (for example, taking a shower, brushing your teeth, drinking coffee, cuddling with your pet), use it as an opportunity to build your attention by really focusing on the activity.

What daily activity could you use to practice mindfulness?

Meditation

Meditation is a formal way to practice mindfulness and has been shown to be a powerful training tool for attention (Norris et al. 2018). There are various types of meditation practice. For example, breath meditation involves being mindful of your breath for a certain time period. When you practice meditation regularly, you will find that you can meditate for longer periods of time—this means your attention is improving! There are many meditation practices online with guided verbal instructions, including body scan meditations of different lengths. Start with short meditations (five to ten minutes) and build from there over time.

Improving Memory

Psychosis impacts each of the three steps involved in memory: encoding (receiving information and preparing it for storage), storage (storing the information in your brain), and retrieval (retrieving the information from your brain). This process is illustrated in the diagram below.

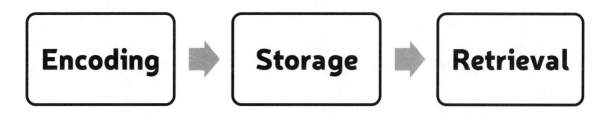

You process and store information in your memory either automatically or with effort. There are several ways to improve your memory, including the following strategies, which are helpful for the encoding process (Caretti et al. 2007):

- **Involve several senses.** If you are trying to remember a short grocery list, for example, you can read the items on paper out loud. You are processing the information visually (by reading the information) and auditorily (by hearing yourself saying the list out loud). Perhaps you also picture the items in your mind while reading them out loud. Can you imagine tasting and smelling the objects as well? Of course, this strategy is easier to use when trying to remember concrete items, like objects (such as pens, apples, and stars).

- **Rehearse and repeat.** Rehearsal, or repeating something several times, will help you remember a list of items or words. Studying for an exam? Flashcards will help you learn the information and can be taken anywhere.

- **Make associations.** Having difficulty remembering people's names? The next time you are introduced to someone, pay attention to their name and repeat it (for example, "It's nice to meet you, Tom."). Then, try to associate their name with an image. Perhaps Tom looks like Tom Hanks or a different Tom you know.

- **Alliterate.** Using alliteration can also aid memory. After meeting Tom, you note, *Tom is tall.*

- **Acronyms are awesome!** Tom is the Only Merman (now picture Tom as a merman). Do you need to remember several items to pick up from the store? Perhaps the items are spinach, milk, oranges, shampoo, and gum. Can you make a sentence from the first letter of each item? Write it down below:

  _____

  _____

- **Self-talk.** As you are performing a task, repeat the steps out loud. This will help you learn and remember the task. You can try this out by looking up instructions for yoga poses. Choose one to practice and read the instructions aloud as you move your body into downward dog, child's pose, tree pose, or warrior II.

- **Personalize the information.** You will have an easier time remembering material the deeper you process it. Reading this text, for example, will be more memorable if you engage in the exercises and apply them to your life. Highlight the skills you want to practice and remember. Try them out and see how they work for you (or not). Reflect on your experiences and write them down. In other words, actively engage with the material!

- **Summarize.** As you are reading this text or any other book, article, or piece of writing, another way to actively engage with the material is to summarize the ideas located in the text. If you are reading a fiction book, you can summarize what happened in each chapter, perhaps out loud to someone else or by writing it down. If someone gives you directions, summarize what they tell you to make sure you got it right.

Improving Processing Speed

You can improve your processing speed, or the time it takes you to process information and react or respond to it (for example, when answering a question), by improving other cognitive abilities. You can also practice tasks repeatedly until they become automatic and ingrained in your muscle memory. Typing is a good example of how practice can lead to improved speed. Here is how Lily improved her processing speed at work:

> On my first day working at a cafe, I was overwhelmed with the information I had to take in, including how to make twelve different kinds of sandwiches. The lunch hour was especially intense. I thought about calling in and quitting, rather than going back. My sister encouraged me to stick with it and offered to practice making sandwiches with me—we made a lot of sandwiches together. With repeated practice, I was able to make each sandwich correctly and quickly.

Like learning an instrument, practicing skills is often the best way to improve performance. Visualization is also an effective tool that can improve performance. Multiple studies have demonstrated the positive impact of visualization on athletic performance, as well as on decreasing anxiety and improving self-confidence (Jose and Joseph 2018). If you find yourself in a similar situation to Lily, practice the skills you need to succeed, both in person and in your mind. You can also set time limits and work toward improving your speed on a given task.

Improving Executive Functioning

The following exercises will assist you with improving your executive functioning, an important set of skills that includes planning and decision making. Executive functioning plays a key role in helping us reach our goals.

Decision Making

Making a pros and cons list is one tool that can assist you with decision making. Even though it is a common tool, we often don't take the time to sit down and write down the pros and cons of a decision we are struggling with. This is unfortunate because making such lists is very helpful with organizing our thoughts. If you are struggling with a decision, use the space below to write the pros and cons of choosing one option. Then, write the pros and cons of another option. Put a star next to items with a lot of significance. When weighing the pros and cons of a particular choice, sometimes the significance of one outweighs several items in the other column.

Decision you need to make: _____

_____

Option 1: _____

Pros	Cons

Option 2: _____

Pros	Cons

Planning

What is one of your goals? Similar to writing down the pros and cons of a decision, an underutilized skill that is helpful for planning is to list each step of the process. It can be overwhelming to think about achieving a long-term goal. By planning and organizing the steps toward your goal, you can track your progress and stay motivated. In the spaces below, identify each step needed to accomplish an important goal.

Your goal: _____

Step (what needs to be accomplished)	Timeline
1.	
2.	
3.	
4.	
5.	
6.	
7.	
8.	
9.	
10.	

Problem Solving

Effective problem solving is an extremely useful skill. It usually includes the following steps:

1. Identify the problem (be specific).

2. Brainstorm possible solutions.

3. Evaluate the solutions.

4. Choose one to try (or a combination of solutions).

5. Evaluate the outcome.

Can you think of an acronym for I-B-E-C-E to help you remember these five steps (for example, "I believe every cat is entitled," or "Introverted bees eat celery every day")?

_____

See how Casey used problem solving to address a specific problem:

Casey had not been on a date in several years. She felt depressed and lonely. Recently, she started working out at the gym three times a week. She also began volunteering at the local humane shelter. She felt ready to meet people to potentially date but did not know where to start. Her peer specialist, Bo, suggested that they approach this as a problem to be solved. They went through the problem-solving process together.

Identify the problem:

I'm anxious about dating again. It's been a long time. I don't feel comfortable making small talk with people. I also don't know where to meet people. My friend Tabitha met her partner online. But I don't know how I feel about that.

Bo pointed out that there are potentially two problems to work on here: (1) feeling uncomfortable making small talk with people (or having conversations in general) and (2) difficulty finding ways to meet new people.

Casey decided that she wanted to work on the first problem before working on the second one.

Brainstorm possible solutions:

Together, they came up with the following solutions:

1. Practice making small talk with people I know (Bo, Mom, Tabitha).

2. Practice making small talk with people I don't know but who seem friendly (for example, a barista, a supermarket clerk, a few people at the drop-in center).

3. Enroll in a social-skills training class.

4. Write down a list of my interests and questions that I could ask someone I am trying to get to know.

5. Ask my psychiatrist for an anti-anxiety medication.

6. Practice deep breathing exercises.

7. Ask Tabitha for her advice on how she was able to talk to her partner, Matt, at first.

Evaluate the solutions:

Casey immediately eliminated #2 ("too nerve-wracking"), #3 ("too time-consuming"), #5 ("I don't want to take another medication"), and #6 ("It won't help me actually talk to someone"). She also eliminated #7 ("Tabitha is a lot more outgoing than me.").

Choose one to try (or a combination of solutions):

Casey decided she wanted to start with #4 and then implement #1. She figured she could combine these two solutions since they worked well together.

Evaluate the outcome:

After practicing making small talk with people whom she felt comfortable with, Casey felt more confident about her ability to engage in conversation with others. She said she was ready to try #2 next!

Choose a problem to solve in the table below. Make sure the problem you identify is specific and solvable. A blank template is located on the website for this book: http://www.newharbinger.com/53394.

Identify the problem.

Brainstorm possible solutions.

Evaluate the solutions.

Choose one to try (or a combination of solutions).

Evaluate the outcome.

Improving Social Cognition

The following set of exercises is helpful in improving your social cognition, which includes skills that help you better understand other people and be more effective in your relationships.

Exercise #1

Write about a recent conflict you had with someone. What happened? What were you thinking during the conflict? How did you feel? What did you do?

_____

_____

_____

_____

_____

_____

_____

_____

_____

_____

_____

_____

_____

Now take the perspective of the other person in your conflict. Write about the same conflict, but from the point of view of the other person. What happened? What might they have been thinking? How might they have been feeling? What did they do?

_____

_____

_____

_____

_____

_____

_____

_____

_____

_____

_____

_____

_____

Exercise #2

Lots of stories and poems are told from unusual perspectives, providing readers with a different view of the original story (for example, the movie *Maleficent* is an alternate telling of *Sleeping Beauty*).

In the space below, write a poem or short story from the point of view of someone unexpected, perhaps a famous person or character, a misunderstood family member, or your younger or older self.

_____

_____

_____

_____

_____

_____

_____

_____

_____

_____

_____

_____

_____

_____

Other ways to improve social cognition include:

- reading literary fiction

- playing role-playing games

- watching movies and shows

- asking others about their thoughts and feelings at different points in their lives, in different situations, and other scenarios.

Summary

Psychosis can negatively impact several important cognitive abilities, including attention, memory, processing speed, executive functioning, and social cognition. These cognitive symptoms can make it harder to reach your short-, medium-, and long-term goals. In this chapter, we included exercises to help you improve your cognitive abilities or thinking skills. Just like building a muscle, repeatedly practicing the skills in this chapter will help strengthen your cognitive abilities so cognitive symptoms have less of an impact on your life. Next, we turn our attention to overcoming the negative symptoms of psychosis that often accompany these cognitive difficulties.

CHAPTER 7.

Overcoming "Negative Symptoms" and Finding Your Motivation

In this chapter, we explore "negative symptoms" and how to overcome them to help you get moving on your recovery journey. While often not as distressing as "positive symptoms," such as voices and paranoia, negative symptoms can be quite debilitating, as they were for Sam:

> When I was in the hospital, I didn't do much—there really wasn't much to do. My parents told me to just work on getting better. For me, this meant taking meds and sleeping a lot. When I went home, I still didn't feel like doing much of anything. I stopped taking showers and cleaning up after myself. My counselor thought I was depressed, but I didn't really feel sad, or anything really. My psychiatrist told me I was suffering from "negative symptoms" and encouraged me to push myself to do things. "Sure," I said, "I'll try." People don't realize how hard it is to do things when you lack motivation.

What Are Negative Symptoms?

Negative symptoms are thought to be a key feature of psychosis and are typically described as consisting of the following symptoms (known as the "five As"):

- **Affective flattening**—reduced expression of emotions (for example, smiling and laughing less, not showing your emotions as much on your face)

- **Alogia**—talking less than usual, not saying a lot in social situations

- **Avolition**—decreased motivation

- **Asociality**—reduced social activity or social engagement

- **Anhedonia**—loss of pleasure

Negative symptoms are often confused with depression because they appear very similar to each other. When we feel depressed, we can feel shut down and unmotivated to get out of bed or do much of anything. However, while depression is associated with feelings of sadness and guilt, as well as suicidal thoughts, negative symptoms are associated with feelings of apathy and reduced suicide risk (Grover et al. 2022).

Although you may not feel distressed, negative symptoms may dramatically reduce your quality of life and ability to function in various contexts, such as at school or work, in your relationships, and in your activities of daily living (Ho et al. 1998; Rabinowitz et al. 2012). In fact, negative symptoms are more likely than positive symptoms (voices and paranoia) to lead to both a lower quality of life and difficulty functioning (Rabinowitz et al. 2012). Negative symptoms are also associated with—and made worse by—cognitive difficulties (Harvey et al. 2006) and do not typically respond well to medications (Alemon et al. 2017). Approximately 60 percent of people diagnosed with schizophrenia experience negative symptoms (Bobes et al. 2010; Correll and Schooler 2020). Yet these symptoms are often overlooked and go untreated. When was the last time you were asked about your level of motivation to engage in your hobbies or if you have lost interest in other people? Have you noticed a change in your energy level or the pleasure you experience in life since you first experienced psychosis? If so, the good news is that you can use strategies to improve your negative symptoms so you can start to feel more engaged and connected with the world.

Self-Assessment

For each statement below, answer "yes," if you mostly agree with the statement. Answer "no," if you mostly disagree.

	Yes/No
People have a hard time guessing how I feel.	
I tend to speak in a monotone.	
I usually answer questions with only a few words.	
It takes too much effort to explain things to other people.	
I don't really see the point in socializing.	
I feel distant from other people.	
I don't feel motivated to do much of anything.	
My goals don't seem that important to me.	

	Yes/No
Nothing really excites me anymore.	
I'm not looking forward to much.	

If you answered "yes" to any of the questions above, you may be experiencing negative symptoms (the more yeses, the more negative symptoms you may be experiencing). You may even think, *So what?* Or *I don't really care…* This is also consistent with experiencing negative symptoms! It is not unusual for loved ones to be bothered more by your negative symptoms than you are. You, or others, may even refer to yourself as "lazy," not understanding that certain behaviors, including not taking regular showers, are a product of your psychosis or related to medication side effects and attempts to reduce other aspects of psychosis, such as voices. They do not reflect a deficiency in you as a human being or a character flaw. Negative symptoms are quite common for people who experience psychosis—and can be improved upon.

Talk to Your Psychiatric Provider

Even if you are not particularly bothered by how you feel (or what you do not feel), there is still a good chance that you do not want to continue living in this state. If you are taking psychiatric medications, it may be helpful to visit your psychiatric provider and explore ways to reduce the negative side effects that come with antipsychotic and mood stabilizing medications, including feeling tired, sedated, and emotionally numb, or experiencing excessive drooling. This may mean a reduction or changes in your medication.

It is also possible that you are depressed rather than, or in addition to, experiencing negative symptoms. Your psychiatric provider can help differentiate between the two and may adjust your medications accordingly. In the remainder of this chapter, we focus on some of the cognitive and behavioral strategies you can implement in your life to feel more alive and engaged with the world around you. These strategies are helpful for both negative and depressive symptoms (we will focus more on depression in chapter 8).

Defeatist and Other Unhelpful Beliefs

Defeatist beliefs—believing you are going to fail before you even try—contribute to the development and worsening of negative symptoms (Grant and Beck 2009; Luther et al. 2016; Pillny et al. 2020). Changing these beliefs (and the behavior associated with them) will help you get more involved in life, *feel* better, and reach your goals. In addition to low expectations for success, low expectations for pleasure (*I'm not going to enjoy myself, so why bother?*) and acceptance by others (*No one there will want to talk with me.*) can contribute to disengagement from the outside world. Below are some examples of beliefs that you may hold. Make a checkmark next to the statements you agree with.

- ☐ *It is not worth trying because I will fail.*
- ☐ *It is terrible to fail at something.*
- ☐ *I have failed more than most people.*
- ☐ *I am unlikely to enjoy new activities.*
- ☐ *It is not worth the effort to try new things.*
- ☐ *I am unlikely to be accepted by others.*
- ☐ *I cannot tolerate rejection.*

The more items you checked, the more likely you are to hold defeatist or other unhelpful beliefs that may be holding you back from engaging in potentially rewarding activities, such as going to a party, meeting new people, or applying for a job.

The following questions will help you identify both helpful and unhelpful (possibly defeatist) beliefs.

Exercise #1. A Recent Success

1. Identify a recent accomplishment.

_____

_____

2. Describe how you were able to accomplish this task.

_____

_____

_____

_____

_____

_____

3. What did you learn from this experience? About yourself? Your abilities?

_____

_____

_____

_____

_____

_____

_____

Exercise #2. An Avoided Task

1. Now identify an important task that you are avoiding (perhaps a task associated with a goal you identified in chapter 2).

_____

_____

2. When you think about performing this task, what emotions do you feel? What thoughts come up?

_____

_____

_____

_____

_____

3. Do these thoughts relate to any beliefs you have about yourself, others, or your future?

_____

_____

_____

_____

_____

_____

_____

Alternative (and More Helpful) Beliefs

Defeatist beliefs are likely protective in some way (for example, against failure, rejection, or disappointment). However, they also hold us back from reaching our goals. We have included alternative beliefs to consider below. We encourage you to consider these alternative beliefs and, like a coat, try them on; see how they feel. It may take some time, as well as new experiences, to fully inhabit them. You may also already have alternative beliefs (perhaps identified in the first exercise above) that help you overcome any resistance or roadblock that you are experiencing in your life.

Defeatist or Other Unhelpful Belief	Alternative and More Helpful Belief
It is not worth trying because I will fail.	It's not guaranteed that I will fail. Also, even if I do fail, I can still learn something from the experience.
It is terrible to fail at something.	Failure is a part of life. It does not reflect my worth as a person. It's definitely something that I can handle.
I have failed more than most people.	I don't need to compare myself with others. I also don't know what most people have been through.
I am unlikely to enjoy new activities.	I won't know if I like something until I try it.
It is not worth the effort to try new things.	It may be worth the effort—I'll find out!

I am not likely to be accepted by others.	*I may find people I like and want to get to know better.*
I cannot tolerate rejection.	*Rejection is painful, but it's part of life and does not mean anything about my value. I can tolerate it, even if I don't like it.*

For the beliefs you identified in exercise #2, can you come up with alternative and more helpful beliefs? Write them in the boxes below.

Defeatist or Other Unhelpful Belief	Alternative and More Helpful Belief

The "I Need to Feel Like It" Myth

We are constantly driven to make decisions based on how we feel: *What do you feel like eating for dinner? What kind of movie do you feel like watching? Do you feel like going out today? Do you feel satisfied with your job? Do you feel in love with your partner?* Our emotions are very helpful in guiding our behavior and letting us know what we value. "Negative emotions," or unpleasant emotions, such as sadness, anger, jealousy, and resentment, can also signal the need for change. However, we learn quite early in life that we cannot *always* follow our emotions, especially if we want to live in harmony with others. If we want to keep our job, we need to show up, regardless of our lack of sleep the night before. We may also choose to make sacrifices in the short term (for example, being thrifty and saving money) to achieve a long-term goal (such as purchasing a desired item). If you find yourself using any of the following phrases on a regular basis, you may be falling for the "I need to feel like it" myth:

"I will do it when I feel like it…"

"I don't have the motivation…"

"I'm too tired…"

Instead, see what happens when you focus on the following belief: *I don't have to feel like doing something in order to do it*, or *I can choose to do* _____ *(insert valued action), even if I don't feel like it.*

Building Awareness: How would your life be different if you were not driven (as much) by your emotions and energy level? What would you do differently?

_____

_____

_____

_____

_____

_____

_____

Changing Your Behavior

While it would be wonderful to have the motivation to do the things we need to or want to do, sometimes we simply don't have it. In other words, we may need to get moving, even if we don't feel like it, to accomplish our goals. We may, in fact, find that the motivation comes later. This is illustrated with a popular strategy you may have heard of: the "five-minute rule." It's simple yet effective. Here are the directions:

1. Choose something that you have been avoiding, or that you typically avoid doing, even though you know it would be helpful to you. For example, cleaning your bathroom or calling a friend.

2. Commit to engaging in the avoided activity for five minutes. You can quit after the five minutes are up. Forgo any judgments or self-criticisms. In fact, plan on congratulating yourself at the end of the five minutes.

3. Do the activity for five minutes. Once the five minutes are up, you can either continue with the activity or quit. It's up to you!

You may find that after five minutes, you don't want to stop. You can make this the "ten-minute rule" over time or the "fifteen-minute rule." It's consistent with the laws of physics. It takes effort to overcome inertia and get moving. Once you are in motion, however, you start to build momentum until it takes effort to stop.

Another strategy for changing your behavior is to schedule activities into your day or week (you can find templates on the website for this book: http://www.newharbinger.com/53394). Write an activity in your daily or weekly schedule that helps you get closer to one of your goals. Then complete the task on the assigned day and time. It's important to check-in later to see how it went.

If you completed your task, congratulate yourself (you could also reward yourself with a desired item or activity)! If you didn't complete your task, identify what got in the way and ways to overcome these obstacles. Then, try again with the solutions you came up with. Sometimes you may find that you need to work on the obstacles you identified before you can proceed with your chosen behavior. This is totally normal and part of the process of change. You may also find that the task you decided on was too much to take on at this time. It's 100 percent okay to set a more realistic goal to work on or give yourself a break.

Getting Connected

Although we have been talking about doing things even if we don't feel like it, this does not mean that feelings are not important or that we should discard how we feel. Our emotions are a big part of our experiences, so it can be disheartening to feel like our emotions are diminished because of medications or for other reasons. Perhaps you have just started feeling disconnected from everything, or perhaps you have been feeling this way for a long time. Whatever the case, we encourage you to try the following exercises to feel more connected to yourself and the world around you—to feel more alive.

Feeling connected to nature is associated with happiness, vitality, and life satisfaction (Capaldi et al. 2014). There are many ways to become more connected to nature, but the best way to feel more connected to nature is to spend time in nature. This means going outside and sitting in a garden, walking on a patch of grass (with bare feet), going for a walk in a forest, and observing squirrels or other wildlife. Instead of being distracted by your phone, you could leave it at home or only use it to take pictures of what you find beautiful or interesting. While it is helpful to live in naturally beautiful places, you don't need go to the best-rated park in your city or town. In fact, the next exercise involves choosing something small in nature to focus on.

Exercise #1. Mindful Observation of a Natural Item

1. Choose one natural item to focus on for the next five minutes. This item could be a small houseplant or a leaf on the sidewalk. It could be a broken branch or a handful of dirt. Pick an item that you can get close to (within two or three feet) so you can note the details of the object.

2. Focus all your attention on this item. Use your senses to notice everything you can about it. What does it look and smell like? What are its various textures and hues? You may be the only person who has ever looked closely at this item and really appreciated it for its uniqueness. Acknowledge the item's limited and temporary existence.

3. Notice any thoughts, images, and memories that come up as you are observing this object. Notice that you are a breathing, living being who is interacting with a natural object at this exact moment in time. So many things have happened in your life to lead you to this moment. The object has also perhaps grown or traveled to end up here with you. This is a moment of connection to be savored.

You can complete this exercise with other natural objects, such as insects and animals, and even with another person!

Exercise #2. Connecting to Yourself

Write down a memory of a time when you were a child and experiencing strong feelings—either positive or negative feelings. If you have a lot of childhood trauma, choose a memory that is not overwhelming or too intense. What were you experiencing at the time? Can you recall who was there, what your environment was like, and what you were feeling in your body?

_____

_____

_____

_____

_____

_____

_____

Now choose a different memory from when you were older, perhaps in your late teens, again when you were experiencing strong feelings. What were they? Do you remember what it felt like in your body at that time? What sort of things you were interested in and passionate about? Write them down below, in addition to what you remember from that moment.

_____

_____

_____

_____

_____

_____

_____

_____

Choose a recent memory of a time when you were experiencing strong feelings. Again, write them down and describe what was going on at the time. What thoughts were you having? What were you feeling? What were you doing?

_____

_____

_____

_____

_____

_____

_____

_____

Take some time to reflect on how you have changed over time. Can you appreciate the similarities and differences between your various selves at different points in your life? Let go of any judgments you have about yourself at any point in your life. Take a few moments to appreciate the progression of your life over time and all of the experiences you have been through as a human being.

Summary

Negative symptoms, including a lack of motivation and feelings of apathy, are often overlooked in the treatment of psychosis. Yet, they are important to address if they are negatively impacting your quality of life or functioning. Defeatist beliefs may be contributing to less engagement with your environment. Identifying the beliefs that are getting in the way of working toward your goals is the first step toward overcoming them. You can change your beliefs as well as your behavior to engage more with others, work toward your goals, and feel better overall. You can also practice mindfulness to feel a deeper sense of connection to yourself and the world around you. These exercises are also helpful to overcome feelings of depression, which we will explore further in the next chapter.

CHAPTER 8.

Managing Mania, Depression, and Suicidal Ideation

If you are struggling with depression right now, we wish we could take the burden from you and set it aside, even for a short period of time. Depression can permeate your whole being and make you believe that you are not deserving of love and acceptance—nothing could be further from the truth. Yet if you are depressed, this may be difficult to believe because your mind keeps focusing on the negative. Depression is also associated with feeling sad, irritable, apathetic, guilty, hopeless, and suicidal. You may experience significant changes in your appetite and sleep patterns while struggling with feelings of exhaustion. Taken together, the symptoms of depression can make it hard to get out of bed, let alone function. This is why depression is considered a serious mental illness. In 2021, approximately 8.3 percent of adults in the United States experienced an episode of depression, including 18.6 percent of people between the ages of eighteen and twenty-five (Substance Abuse and Mental Health Services Administration 2021). If you experience depression, you are not alone, even though it may feel like it.

Consider Maya's story:

> I started hearing voices telling me to kill myself as a teenager. I think I was fourteen. By then, I had already been depressed for a few years and had started cutting myself just to feel better. I literally felt like my life and everything in it was suffocating me. I wanted to escape from it all. I wanted to escape from my body and the pain that seemed to live inside of me. All I could think about was dying and being free. My voices were just saying what I thought everyone else wanted to say to me but didn't have the guts to—that I would be better off dead.

In this chapter, we discuss coping skills for depression, building on the skills from chapter 7 (overcoming negative symptoms). Then, we talk about preventing mania, which may come before or after a depressive episode. Finally, we discuss how to cope with suicidal thinking. Whether you are dealing with depression, mania, or suicidal thinking, we offer you support and encouragement. Remember that you didn't always feel this way, and you won't feel this way forever. There are things that you can do to improve how you feel both in the short and long term.

Interventions for Depression

When you experience depression, everything seems slowed down. You may try to self-medicate with caffeine, only to crash later. If you find that you have pulled back from activities you used to enjoy, it is important to start engaging in those activities again, even if you don't feel like it. Activities that increase your sense of mastery and pleasure tend to improve your mood (Beck 1979). These are not the same thing, since mastery tends to be associated with a sense of accomplishment (such as accomplishing a goal), whereas pleasure tends to be mostly physical (such as eating ice cream) and involves your senses. Some activities increase both your sense of mastery and pleasure (such as going on a hike somewhere beautiful) and may be especially rewarding. Rather than being a passive recipient to how you feel, engaging in such activities is taking an active stance in learning how to change how you feel. You are taking charge of your mental health and doing things to feel better, one day at a time.

Increasing Mastery and Pleasure

In the lists below, circle the challenging and pleasurable activities you are willing to try to improve your mood. Then, engage in these activities and notice if they impact how you feel. Rate your level of sadness before and after the activity (or focus on another symptom of depression, such as feeling tired or having a lack of energy). Then note which activities seem to have the most impact on your depressive symptoms. This list is just a starting point, so make sure to continue adding activities over time in both categories.

Challenging Activities	Pleasurable Activities
Solve a crossword puzzle	Read a book or magazine
Fold origami	Take a shower or bath
Learn to play an instrument	Walk in the forest
Work on your handstand	Listen to loud music
Sketch a favorite place	Eat your favorite food
Write a poem	Paint your nails
Memorize a poem	Talk to a friend
Teach someone a skill that you know well	Sunbathe
Learn about a new subject	Watch a movie
Put a puzzle together	Watch cat videos
Work on solving a real-world problem	Write in your journal
Do push-ups and crunches	Try on different outfits
Learn a new recipe to cook	Pet a cat or dog
Teach your pet a new trick	Watch a new show
Make a collage or vision board (with pictures representing your goals and values)	Hum or sing out loud
	Play video games
Write a review of a movie or book	Have sex or masturbate
Write someone a handwritten letter	Engage in aromatherapy
Make a dating profile online	Take pictures with your camera or phone
Other: _____	Other: _____
Other: _____	Other: _____

Dialing In Your Compassionate Figure

Practicing self-compassion is an especially powerful skill that can alleviate depression, and one that you can cultivate with time and practice. It is helpful to have a wise, compassionate figure or voice that you can come back to. Perhaps this is someone in your life who knows you and accepts you completely. It could also be a spiritual figure, such as an all-loving god. It could be a character in a movie that struck you as particularly kind and generous or the imagined voice of an affectionate and loyal pet (if only they could speak!). Once you have identified your compassionate figure, take a moment to envision them and feel comforted by their presence.

Now, from their perspective, write a letter to yourself, addressing your feelings of depression and all the pain that you've been experiencing (Neff n.d.). Imagine that this compassionate figure knows you better than anyone—all your strengths and weaknesses, dreams, and insecurities—they see you fully and accept you *as you are*. They love you, absolutely, and they know just how much you are hurting, and it hurts them to see you hurting so much. They want you to be able to see what they see: you, in all your complexity, a human being who is worthy of the utmost care and compassion. What might they want you to really understand about yourself and your situation?

Dear (your name) _____,

I know that you are suffering right now…

_____

_____

_____

_____

_____

_____

_____

With love and compassion,

(your compassionate figure)_____

The Power of Mania

After experiencing a depressive episode, you may experience a manic episode, or vice versa. Consider Rosie's story:

> I was in graduate school when I had my first manic episode. I remember being under a lot of stress at the time. I was taking classes, teaching a class, conducting research, and trying to keep a long-distance relationship from imploding. At first, I was mostly worried about keeping up with everything. And then I started sleeping less and barely eating. Soon I had lots of ideas. I thought they were brilliant at the time, but now I look back and can see that I wasn't thinking straight. I thought I was going to win the Nobel Prize. I spent a week conducting experiments and writing down all my ideas. By the end of it, I wasn't making any sense at all. I felt so humiliated when I came down from my mania and realized that I was in a psych ward. It felt like I had fallen off a cliff.

In many ways, *mania* is the opposite of depression. When you are manic, you feel invincible and are filled with energy. You may act impulsively, such as spending all your money or starting or ending relationships suddenly. If you experience mania, you may also experience hallucinations and delusions while manic. Experiencing mania can be intense and thrilling. It can feel like a superpower. Unfortunately, it can also be a destructive force in your life, like a tornado, leading to hospitalization and feelings of regret. Common signs of mania include:

- racing thoughts

- talking and moving fast

- having a lot more energy

- sleeping very little or not at all

- feeling elated

- feeling easily frustrated

- acting impulsively, including engaging in risky behavior (for example, substance abuse)

- feeling a lot more interested in sex.

The diagnoses of bipolar I disorder and schizoaffective disorder, bipolar type, are associated with symptoms of mania. If you have been given either of these diagnoses, there is a good chance you have been prescribed a mood stabilizer in addition to an antipsychotic medication. Coming down from mania may lead to depression and feelings of hopelessness, especially if you have done or said things that go against your values, character, or better judgment while manic. *Hypomania*, a less severe form of mania, can still be problematic but is not as debilitating.

Prevent Mania from Reoccurring

You can often prevent mania from reoccurring by following a healthy routine, managing your stress, knowing your triggers, and intervening appropriately when you start to notice your warning signs. We talked about setting up a healthy routine in chapter 3. Getting enough sleep is especially important in preventing mania, which means going to sleep and waking up around the same time and developing positive sleep habits (such as winding down in the evening and avoiding screen time before bed). It is also helpful to be active during the day and give your body time to relax at night. Taking your medications at the same time every day is also part of maintaining a healthy routine. Talk to your psychiatric provider if you feel overly sedated during the day and are having trouble going to sleep at night because the timing of your medications may be adjusted to help with this.

Manage Your Stress

Some stress is helpful, as it can be motivating. Too much stress, however, can lead to burnout (of course, sometimes we don't have a choice, and we must deal with situations we have little control over). There is a lot of research that suggests too much stress is terrible for our health, especially when we are chronically stressed-out (Yaribeygi et al. 2017). Too much stress can also trigger a manic episode. Take a moment to consider your responsibilities and challenges. Do you have the resources and skills to manage your responsibilities and overcome the challenges that you are experiencing? If your answer is not an immediate yes, you are likely under a significant amount of stress! You can change your level of stress by either (1) finding ways to reduce the responsibilities and challenges you are facing or (2) increasing your resources and relevant skills. Consider Reggie's decision:

> I chose to go from working full time to part time. It wasn't an easy decision to make. For so long, work really defined me. It was the source of my self-worth. I was good at my job as a nurse. I had a decent income and a few supportive coworkers. But I think work-related stress is what led to my most recent episode of mania, which I am still recovering from. I ended up losing my apartment while I was hospitalized, so now I live with my sister. It's not ideal, but I like her company, and I am paying a lot less for rent and utilities. I don't want to live with her forever, but for now, I can afford to cut back on my hours and focus on my health.

Take a moment to check in with yourself and your level of stress lately. Is this a good amount of stress to experience? How does your body feel? If you are experiencing a lot of stress, is there anything that you can do to reduce the amount of stress in your life?

_____

_____

_____

_____

Doing the Exact Opposite

"Opposite action" is a skill where you do the exact opposite of what your emotions are telling you to do (Linehan 2015). So, if you are depressed and want to isolate, you push yourself to seek out company instead. The idea behind opposite action is to change how you feel through your actions (your emotions will likely follow!). If you are starting to feel hypomanic or even manic, you may want to socialize, go shopping, or engage in exciting activities. If you notice these feelings and urges coming up in your body, _do the exact opposite_. Rest. Listen to calming music. Turn down the lights and reduce your stimulation. Stop scrolling through your phone. What other activities can you do to slow down?

_____

_____

_____

_____

Identify Your Triggers and Warning Signs

Whether you have had one manic episode or several, it is important to recognize your triggers and warning signs so you can prevent another manic episode from wreaking havoc on your life. _Triggers_ refer to anything that can bring on a manic episode, like physical illness or a stressful life event (such as starting a new job, moving, or getting married). You may also notice that seasonal changes are associated with episodes of mania or depression (Fellinger et al. 2019; Geoffroy et al. 2013). Antidepressants can also trigger mania (Tondo et al. 2010). *Warning signs*, meanwhile, are internal changes that may signal you are about to experience a manic episode. For example, you may notice that your sense of humor becomes more biting or that you become more social and want to go out more. Do you remember what preceded your last manic episode? Building your awareness includes understanding your triggers and warning signs so you know what to look out for. You will list these on your relapse prevention plan, which you will create in chapter 10.

Stop Mania in Its Tracks

If you recognize that you are heading toward a manic episode, how do you put on the breaks and change course? Possible interventions include the following:

- Ask your psychiatric provider to adjust your medication(s)—this could be on a temporary basis until you no longer are experiencing warning signs.

- Talk to your therapist or your peer recovery specialist.

- Seek additional social support from friends and family members.

- Reduce your stress level (for example, take time off work).

- Prioritize sleep and self-care.

- Eliminate caffeine and other stimulating substances.

Even if you have had multiple episodes of mania or hypomania in the past, do not be discouraged! Each setback you experience provides valuable information you can use to improve your relapse prevention plan and intervene more effectively.

Suicide: The Last Resort

Experiencing a depressive or manic episode, or a mix of the two, increases your risk of suicide significantly (Sher et al. 2001). Psychosis is also associated with an increased risk of suicidal thoughts, suicide attempts, and death by suicide (Yates et al. 2019). It makes sense to think of suicide as an option when you are experiencing deep and prolonged suffering. Too often, however, it may seem like the only solution or the best one when it really is a last resort (and we would argue that there are always other options and hope for things getting better). Suicide is permanent and leaves behind further pain and suffering.

Suicidal Ideation Is Not the Problem

Being able to solve problems effectively is perhaps one of the most important skills in this section. The problem is not that you are experiencing suicidal thinking. Suicide is one possible solution to your problem, which likely has several, if not many, possible solutions that you have not considered or tried yet.

When you think about the reasons you have been suicidal in the past or are currently suicidal, what comes to mind? Possible reasons may include feelings of isolation, loneliness, shame, guilt, or self-hatred. You may feel stuck, like you are a burden to others, or consumed with anger for past wrongs, flooded with what seems like unbearable memories.

_____

_____

_____

_____

_____

If you are feeling hopeless, what are you feeling hopeless about (for example, finding work, finding a romantic partner, finding acceptance)?

_____

_____

_____

If you were recently suicidal or are currently suicidal, what are the top three problems you are trying to solve with suicide?

1. _____

2. _____

3. _____

Consider Arthur's underlying problems:

I've been depressed ever since my wife, Sheila, died two years ago. Her death was sudden and unexpected. I couldn't imagine living without her for the rest of my life. Although I have children and grandchildren, I don't see them very often. I also don't want to be a burden to them. After Sheila died, I stopped going to church because I was angry at God for taking my wife away from me...right after he took my mom away. I also have health issues that make it hard for me to walk or do a lot. It's a lot to deal with.

When Arthur's therapist asked him what was behind his desire to die, he immediately replied, "Missing my wife." Arthur and his therapist brainstormed the following possible solutions to this problem:

- Spending time each day honoring her memory (such as listening to her favorite music, eating her favorite foods, going through pictures of their family) for thirty minutes to an hour.

- Writing her a letter like he used to when they were first dating, telling her about his day.

- Talking about her with his children and grandchildren.

- Focusing on helping animals in some way. She loved animals, and they loved her back.

Arthur decided to try the first option and found that it helped alleviate some of the pain of missing his wife. However, he realized that he still had other problems he wanted to solve, including feelings of loneliness and anger toward God. These problems required additional problem-solving strategies.

After you have identified your primary drivers for suicide, spend some time focusing on just one problem, and complete the steps of problem solving using the boxes below (you can find a template on the website for this book: http://www.newharbinger.com/53394). Focus on one problem at a time so you don't feel too overwhelmed and try to have a realistic view of how long it may take to solve a big problem, such as loneliness. Celebrate small successes and your daily efforts.

Identify the problem.

Brainstorm possible solutions.

Evaluate the solutions.

Choose one to try (or a combination of solutions).

Evaluate the outcome.

Safety Planning

It is important to come up with a safety plan if you are experiencing any suicidal thinking or have in the past. Safety plans save lives (Stanley and Brown 2012). Keep this plan somewhere visible (for example, on your fridge). Before filling out your safety plan, it is important to decrease your access to means of suicide. Do you have access to any lethal means or ways to kill yourself? This could include owning a firearm or having access to certain medications. If so, are you willing to get rid of these means? If you are not willing to get rid of them, can you give them to another person in the meantime (until at least you are feeling better)? You are a lot less likely to kill yourself if you simply don't have the means.

Below is a template for a safety plan that we encourage you to fill out, preferably with someone you trust, such as your therapist or a peer support specialist (you can download a worksheet from http://www.newharbinger.com/53394).

Warning signs: (Signs that you may start to feel more suicidal.)

_____

_____

_____

_____

_____

What to focus on instead: (What can you distract yourself with? Include activities that you can do on your own and activities that you can do with other people.)

_____

_____

_____

_____

_____

List your support people and their contact information:

Name	Contact Information
Emergency contacts: 988 Suicide and Crisis Lifeline, Text "TALK" to 741741, 911	

Commit to using this plan if you start to feel suicidal. It is completely okay to reach out for help—it's lifesaving and a sign of wisdom. You are a human being unlike any other human being on this planet. Your life is precious—we mean that truly. We are glad that you are here reading this right now.

Reasons for Living

What are your reasons for living? What keeps you going through the pain and suffering? Write them down! There is no such thing as a "silly" reason to live. Everything matters, including the next season of your favorite TV show, your favorite people, animals, foods and snacks, and places. This list could also be titled "My Favorite Things in Life."

_____

_____

_____

_____

_____

_____

_____

_____

_____

_____

_____

_____

_____

_____

_____

Keep this list with you, perhaps in your wallet or on your bathroom mirror. Add to your list as you are reminded or given more reasons to live and breathe.

This is also an evocative question to explore with other people ("What are your reasons for living?") because many people have not given a lot of consideration to this question.

Creating a Hope Box

Finally, we invite you to create a "hope box" (Berk et al. 2004). This intervention can be very powerful and life-affirming. It also offers you something tangible to look at, feel, touch, and smell (and perhaps taste) when you are feeling hopeless or need reminders that life is worth living. Here are the instructions:

1. Find a box. A shoebox works nicely, but it can be any kind of box that can hold meaningful objects that give you hope.

2. Write "My Hope Box" at the top of your box. Decorate your box. You could use stickers, draw or paint your box, or attach pictures or magazine pages.

3. Put important objects, memories (such as pictures), letters, and items in the box. Include whatever object is meaningful to you. It could be a poem or song lyrics, perhaps a phrase that inspires hope, a book that you strongly resonated with, or chocolate. Maybe it's a compliment that has stuck with you (write it down!).

4. Put your hope box near your bed. When you are feeling hopeless, come back to the objects in your box and hold individual items in your hands for comfort and consideration. Feel the weight of each object. What feelings come up for you?

5. Feel free to change the items in your box over time. What gives you hope may change over time, or perhaps it won't. It may be that you come back to the same things over and over again.

Summary

Depression is painful and relatively common. The same interventions for negative symptoms can be used to help alleviate depression. We recommend engaging in activities that increase your sense of mastery and pleasure and consistently practicing self-compassion. If you have ever experienced a manic or hypomanic episode, know that there are things you can do to decrease the likelihood of experiencing another manic episode, including taking good care of yourself, managing your stress, monitoring your warning signs and triggers, and intervening appropriately. Suicide is a permanent and tragic solution to problems of living. You can address your problems and overcome them—suicide is the last resort. Problem solving is an important skill to practice repeatedly. We strongly believe there is no problem that cannot be overcome with a combination of support, resources, and skills. The next chapter focuses on fighting stigma—a relevant and important topic!

CHAPTER 9

Letting Go of Stigma

None of us are immune to experiencing symptoms of mental illness. In fact, global surveys have revealed that mental health concerns are common. For example, the World Health Organization distributed a survey in twenty-eight countries and found mental health concerns were reported by people in all participating countries, with a lifetime prevalence rate of between 18 to 36 percent (Kessler et al. 2009). Other surveys have estimated that anywhere between 5 to 20 percent of people experience transitory psychotic symptoms (McGrath et al. 2015; Turkington and Spencer 2019). So why does it sometimes feel like discussing our mental health concerns is *taboo*?

What Is Mental Health Stigma?

Mental health *stigma* refers to negatively biased beliefs about people with mental health problems and diagnoses. Oftentimes these beliefs are fueled by misinformation, fear, and prejudice. They harm everyone but are especially harmful to those with mental illness.

Stigmatizing depictions and messages about mental illness can be found in popular culture (such as television, movies, music, books), online message boards, outdated educational materials, and in the language and actions of those around us.

Examples of mental health stigma include:

- Attitudes, such as viewing a person with mental illness as weak, incompetent, immoral, or childlike

- Labels, such as "crazy," "lunatic," or "insane"

- Stereotypes, such as "people with psychosis are dangerous or violent," "psychosis cannot be treated," or "people with psychosis cannot work or have relationships"

- Depictions, such as showing images of people with mental health concerns as disheveled, incoherent, restrained or imprisoned, or portraying psychiatric treatment centers as inhumane prisons with horrid conditions, including "asylum"-themed horror attractions.

Internalized stigma, or *self-stigma*, refers to the process of applying these negative messages to yourself, for example, labeling yourself as "crazy" or telling yourself you will not amount to anything because of your diagnosis. Internalized stigma can leave you feeling ashamed, embarrassed, less-than, or angry at yourself for having psychosis. In some cases, you may even withdraw from your relationships, hobbies, communities, and goals, or feel hopeless about your future.

No one is immune to the impact of stigma. Like a fish growing up surrounded by water, we grow up surrounded by the culture or cultures we were raised in. This includes growing up around stigmatizing messages about others: other people, places, and circumstances. Just as the fish likely does not think much about the water that surrounds it, we often do not stop to reflect on the culture or cultures that surround us, and in turn, do not stop to reflect on how our culture might be impacting us.

The goal of this chapter is to teach you how to identify these toxic beliefs and, if present, ways to combat the harmful effects of stigma.

Building Awareness: Above we listed common examples of stigmatizing messages from Western, specifically American, culture. Are there any other stigmatizing messages about mental illness or psychosis you've encountered from any culture you are a part of?

_____

_____

_____

_____

_____

_____

How Does Stigma Impact You?

Addressing the impact of stigma and self-stigma is a critical part of recovery because research has found that stigma and self-stigma:

- Discourage people from reaching out for help with their symptoms (Xu et al. 2016)

- Hurt self-esteem (Vilhauer 2017; Wood et al. 2017)

- Contribute to voices feeling more powerful, becoming more negative, and happening more frequently (Vilhauer 2017; Wood et al. 2018)

- Lead to episodes of discrimination, for example, being denied employment, housing, or being assaulted or harassed (Brohan and Thornicroft 2010; Compton and Broussard 2009; Albers et al. 2018)

- Contribute to increased isolation or feeling more disconnected from one's community (Vilhauer 2017)

- Make people less likely to follow their treatment plan (Bornheimer et al. 2021)

- Make it feel more difficult for someone to talk about what they are going through with others (Wood et al 2018).

All the above make it harder to recover from psychosis. Imagine your recovery journey is like climbing a mountain. Of course, like any long journey, we can expect natural peaks and valleys, good moments and hard moments, even when we're trying our best. However, each bullet point above is like a rock you pick up along the way and place in your backpack. The more rocks you carry, or the more negative messages you tell yourself about the person you are, the harder the journey will be.

Here's Hal's description of how stigma affected him:

When I first got diagnosed with psychosis, it felt like the elephant in the room for months. No one knew how to talk about it, myself included, so we just didn't. Those early days were lonely and stressful. When I'd think about psychosis, I'd think of people in horror films, either frail and stuck in a straitjacket or out of control and violent. I didn't relate to either of those, but it made me wonder if that would be my future. I worried people would automatically assume I was "crazy." It really took a toll on me. Learning about the diagnosis and getting connected with peer support groups helped a lot. Eventually I, and my friends and family, found it easier to talk about. I got the support I needed and was able to spend more time reconnecting with the parts of life that I love.

Building Awareness: Do you relate to any of the bullet points above? If so, which harmful effects of stigma have impacted you the most?

_____

_____

_____

_____

_____

Recognizing Stigma

To heal the hurtful labels we may have placed on ourselves, we first have to recognize them. Take a moment to think about how you talk about yourself, either to others or privately, in your own mind. Jot down how you would describe yourself:

_____

_____

_____

_____

_____

_____

_____

Do you see any hurtful language in your self-description? If so, take another moment to reflect on where this language might have come from. Again, stigmatizing messages can come from the language and actions of those around us and are often perpetuated by popular culture (such as movies, television, music). Consider Leah's story, below:

> I was raised in a big city, and sometimes when my dad would take my brother and me out for walks, we would see people on the street talking to themselves. Every time we would pass them, my dad would instruct my brother and me not to make eye contact with them. Sometimes he'd tell us they were "crazy," unpredictable, or on drugs. Eventually I felt scared when I would see we were approaching someone who was talking to themselves. As an adult who hears voices, and often responds to those voices, I feel a deep sense of shame from those early experiences. I imagine everyone I pass is thinking the same things my dad and I used to think. It makes me not want to leave the house some days.

Imagine taking a bite of a bagel and swallowing it whole, without chewing. This is like accepting negative feedback and messages automatically, without considering whether it really applies to you or not.

Try not to swallow negative feedback or messages whole. Instead, chew on it for a while, swallow the parts that feel helpful for your recovery journey, and spit out the rest.

Expanding Labels

One label you may have received is a *diagnosis*. Diagnoses are tools. They are used by medical professionals to quickly and concisely communicate a presenting concern and are offered as a way to help people better understand what is happening to them. Diagnoses were never intended to overshadow other parts of your identity. However, if you have ever been labeled "a patient," "schizophrenic," "bipolar," "antisocial," or "borderline," you may relate to feeling like this label defines or follows you.

When a diagnosis or label starts to feel like your predominant or only identity, it can be helpful to reconnect with other parts of yourself. In the box below, write down some other identities you could use to label or describe yourself, for example: "friend," "hard worker," "artist," "Muslim," "son," "daughter," "child," or "parent."

Overcoming the Sting of Stigma

Now that you have learned more about stigma and how it may be impacting you, in the following sections you will focus on ways to challenge stigma's hurtful messages and rebuild what stigma may have taken from you.

Affirmations

If internalized stigma has hurt the way in which you view or talk to yourself, practicing daily affirmations can help you rebuild your self-image and self-esteem.

Below are some sample affirmations. There are also spaces to write your own. To practice, take a few minutes each day to repeat the affirmations out loud to yourself. It is not uncommon for this exercise to feel uncomfortable or insincere at first. That is normal, and those feelings will improve with time. Be gentle and patient with yourself as you try something new.

- "I deserve to feel good about myself."

- "I believe in myself."

- "I'm a good person."

- "I am worthy."

- "I am a work in progress, just like everybody else."

- "I can get through hard times."

- "I am enough."

- "I will give my body and mind the care they deserve."

- "I am resilient."

- Write your own: _____

- Write your own: _____

- Write your own: _____

Identifying Role Models

Psychosis can be an isolating experience, and it can sometimes feel like you are the only person in the world going through it. It is not uncommon for people to feel discouraged and concerned about their future during or immediately after an episode of psychosis. If you find yourself at this point, learning more about people who have achieved great things while also living with symptoms of psychosis may help you see that recovery and success are possible. Take a look at the examples below; these individuals reported experiencing symptoms of psychosis at some point in their life.

John Frusciante (b. 1970) American musician best known for his time in the Red Hot Chili Peppers.	Anthony Hopkins (b. 1937) British Academy Award-winning actor, famous works include *The Silence of the Lambs* and *The Father.*	John Forbes Nash, Jr. (1928–2015) American mathematician who won the Nobel Prize in economics.
Brian Wilson (b. 1942) American musician, singer, songwriter, and record producer who cofounded the Beach Boys.	Mahatma Gandhi (1869–1948) Indian leader who used nonviolent resistance to campaign to free India from British rule.	Lionel Aldridge (1941–1998) American football player who played for the Green Bay Packers and the San Diego Chargers.
Carl Jung (1875–1961) Swiss psychiatrist who founded Analytical Psychology.	Vincent van Gogh (1853–1890) Dutch post-impressionist painter whose famous works include *The Starry Night* and *Bedroom in Arles.*	Charles Dickens (1812–1870) English author whose famous works include *Oliver Twist* and *A Christmas Carol.*
Selena Gomez (b. 1992) American singer, actress, and film producer.	Joan of Arc (c. 1412–1441) Catholic saint and French military leader who led the resistance against the English invasion of France.	Insert Your Own:

(Bailey 2022; Belli 2009; Blumer 2002; Eskenazi 1998; Foreman 1954; Schildkrout 2017; Turkington and Spencer 2019)

Illustrations of the people above are on the website for this book, http://www.newharbinger.com/53394, along with suggestions for activities you can complete to further explore your own strengths and goals.

The Positives of Your Psychosis

What we label as "psychosis" can be found in every culture, in every time period, throughout recorded human history. You may have heard stories of historical figures being visited by angels or hearing muses or have heard people describe how their creativity, spirituality, or personal insights were enhanced and enriched by their psychosis—like some of our examples above!

Jordan et al. (2018) formally explored the question, "What are some of the positive changes a person might experience following an episode of psychosis?" They found that experiencing psychosis contributed to a variety of positive outcomes and helped facilitate personal growth, such as:

- "Helping me clarify my values, and what I want out of life"

- "Feeling stronger, more self-reliant, or more resilient to adversity"

- "Finding a deeper meaning in life"

- "Having a greater sense of self-acceptance and self-understanding"

- "Feeling wiser, more imaginative, more in touch with my feelings, more mature, and more open to new ideas"

- "Feeling more spiritual, or more connected to my religion"

- "Holding a deeper appreciation for the people in my life"

- "Contributing to a desire to help and inspire others."

Take a few moments to reflect on any positive aspects of your psychosis. Do you relate to any of the findings above? Offer as much description as you can of any positives that have come with your psychosis:

_____

_____

_____

_____

_____

_____

Talking About Psychosis with Others and Setting Boundaries

Mental health stigma contributes to misinformation and subsequent misunderstanding around psychosis. This can make it challenging to talk about symptoms with others, as you may fear being rejected, made fun of, or misunderstood.

While it may temporarily relieve anxiety to avoid talking about your psychosis, you run the risk of increasing feelings of anxiety, shame, and loneliness over time. You may even deny yourself important medical care, which can worsen and prolong psychosis.

When you disclose your psychosis and how much detail you offer depends on a number of factors, including the context, how well you know the person, and how emotionally safe you are feeling with them in that moment. There is no one right answer. The most important thing is to find trusted others you can talk to and receive support from.

Building Awareness: What would you want to tell the people in your life about your psychosis? If you've discussed your experiences with the people in your life, how did these conversations go?

_____

_____

_____

_____

_____

_____

_____

Building Assertiveness by Asking for What You Need

Stigma can make you feel small, like you and your needs don't matter. Nothing could be further from the truth. We all need help now and then, and you shouldn't feel ashamed for asking for support during an episode of psychosis. To overcome stigma's impact on how you may be treated as a "mental patient" (even by those with good intentions), it can be useful to assertively ask for what you need from others. *Assertive communication* refers to communication that is both direct and respectful (see chapter 4).

When asking for help from others, first consider *what you need* from them. Many times, loved ones sincerely want to be helpful but sometimes do not know how. Here are some examples of how to ask for what you want or need:

- "I'd like you to just listen to me right now, without offering any advice."

- "I need help with (a specific request)."

- "I need you to offer me reassurance right now (that I am safe, that we're okay, that this isn't real)."

- "I'd like you just to be with me right now. I don't feel like talking."

- "I want to talk about something else that will help me feel less stressed."

- "I want to do something fun."

- "I'd like to get out of the house."

- Write your own: _____

- Write your own: _____

Setting Boundaries

There will be times where you do not feel like discussing your psychosis or need to take time away from responsibilities to engage in self-care and rest. These are good opportunities to practice setting boundaries. Boundaries are the limits we set with ourselves and others. *Healthy boundaries* allow us to take good care of ourselves and nurture the relationships that are important to us. Examples of healthy boundaries include:

- Sharing your personal information with your support system

- Asking for help when you need it

- Taking a break when you need it

- Valuing your own wants and needs, while also remaining open to the wants and needs of others

- Saying no to requests that make you uncomfortable

- Leaving relationships that are abusive

- Respecting other people's boundaries.

Here are some signs your boundaries could be improved:

Your boundaries may be too open if you struggle saying no to others, even when the request makes you uncomfortable; you stay in relationships that are harmful to you; you do not allow yourself breaks or work late hours without compensation; or you behave in ways that do not align with your values (for example, you say you value loyalty, but cheat on your partner).

Your boundaries may be too closed if you do not ask for help when needed; you do not share your thoughts and feelings with others, even if they play an important role in your life (such as a romantic partner, best friend, relative); or you avoid making compromises in your close relationships.

If you feel like your boundaries could be improved, welcome! This is a common therapy goal. The good news is that just like any other skill, developing good boundaries can be achieved with repeated practice.

To practice setting boundaries, first identify what boundaries you would like to work on or change. Examples include "I want to get better at saying no to others," and "I want to feel comfortable taking a mental health day from work if I need one." Brainstorm your ideas below:

_____

_____

_____

_____

_____

Next, when you notice your boundary is being pushed (for example, someone pressuring you to do something you don't want to do), use the situation as an opportunity to practice setting a new boundary. Examples of boundary-language include:

- "I appreciate the offer, but I don't want to do that, or I won't be able to do that."

- "Thanks for asking, but I do not feel like talking about this right now."

- "Please do not use that language to describe me."

- "I am not comfortable with this."

- "Going forward I would appreciate it if you did not talk to me this way."

- "I am happy you're inviting me out, but I am not up for going out right now."

Unfortunately, some people have trouble accepting boundaries. If you are not used to setting boundaries with the people in your life, they may struggle to accept the new boundary you have set—they are just as unfamiliar with it as you are! If this happens, hold your ground and reinforce your boundary. You can even take a break and leave the situation if you need to. Space can give them time to process the new dynamic between you. Below are some ways to reinforce boundaries:

- "I'd appreciate it if you stopped asking me about this."

- "Please do not ask me again."

- "This is not something I will change my mind on."

Connecting with Others and Giving Back

The research is clear: stigma contributes to feeling badly about ourselves, increases episodes of isolation and loneliness, and makes it harder to reach out for help.

Fortunately, there are plenty of compassionate people who refuse to buy into the narrative that mental illness is something to be ashamed of. One powerful way to fight stigma is to connect with these compassionate others. This is especially important when we feel our support system is not currently meeting our emotional, psychological, or social needs.

Here are some psychosis peer support groups that can offer support, encouragement, and community:

- National Alliance of Mental Illness (NAMI)

- Hearing Voices Network

- Intervoice

- Students with Psychosis

- Supportiv

- Schizophrenia and Psychosis Action Alliance

What other identities are important to you? For example, you may wish to connect with others who have the same gender, race, ethnicity, sexuality, religion, or profession, or who share the same hobbies and interests. What are some ways you could connect with people from these communities? Brainstorm ideas below:

_____

_____

_____

_____

_____

_____

_____

_____

_____

_____

Finally, two powerful ways to fight stigma are helping to correct misinformation and giving back to others in need. Check off some the following ways in which you hope to fight stigma going forward:

☐ By talking about my experiences with others

☐ By challenging inaccurate messages that I hear about psychosis

☐ By being a role model for others

☐ By volunteering at a hospital or treatment center

☐ By becoming a peer support specialist

☐ By living my best life

☐ By advocating for human rights

☐ Write your own: _____

☐ Write your own: _____

Summary

Mental health stigma refers to negatively biased beliefs about mental health disorders. You may hear stigmatizing messages about psychosis from the media or people around you. Stigma has the potential to negatively impact your self-esteem and to make you feel less-than or separate from your community. If you are struggling with internalized stigma, try challenging negative beliefs by reciting daily affirmations, identifying role models, and reflecting on the positive aspects of your psychosis. Advocate for your needs by asserting yourself and setting boundaries in a way that feels emotionally safe. Finally, connect with peer support communities and consider sharing your story with others.

Up next is the final chapter of our workbook, "Your Relapse Prevention Plan," in which you will put together everything you have learned thus far into a personalized wellness plan that can help you proactively manage symptoms and prevent a mental health relapse from occurring.

CHAPTER 10

Your Relapse Prevention Plan

You have made it to the final chapter! By now you have learned more about psychosis; have identified your personal strengths, values, and goals; and have practiced coping skills for the many symptoms of psychosis. You've also explored your experiences more closely to better understand what your psychosis may be offering you in terms of personal insight. Moving through this workbook took time, energy, and dedication, but you did it, which is an invaluable act of self-compassion and courage. Congratulations on making it this far. This final chapter will guide you in developing a *relapse prevention plan*, or a plan that puts all you have learned into a guide you can use when you notice your psychosis, depression, or mania worsening or reemerging.

What Is Relapse Prevention?

The term "relapse prevention" refers to all the things you do *proactively* to take care of your mental health and prevent worsening of your symptoms. Taking a proactive approach to mental health care means you are doing small things daily to manage your mental health, such as the topics discussed in chapter 3, and you have a plan in place outlining what you will do when things start to become overwhelming. This is a shift away from *reactive* mental health care, which refers to trying to develop a plan when you are already overwhelmed or in crisis.

The goal of relapse prevention is to minimize the impact symptoms have on your life. We want you to feel like you are living the life you want—not one that feels limited or diminished due to symptoms of psychosis. Go back and revisit your recovery road map. Your goals and values are important. You have the skills to overcome obstacles that get in the way. Preventing a relapse of symptoms will help you move forward on your recovery journey.

In this chapter, you will build a customized relapse prevention plan. Creating your plan will include:

- Identifying what you notice when symptoms feel well managed, versus how they feel when they seem out of your control

- Identifying things that you can do regularly to stay well

- Identifying your triggers (what causes stress or symptoms to worsen) and warning signs (How will you know when things are becoming overwhelming?)

- Identifying what you will do when symptoms feel unmanageable or when you are having a mental health emergency (planning for a crisis)

- Identifying how your support system can help you after a mental health flare-up or crisis.

Learning about yourself and your psychosis is a lifelong process. To honor this process, we ask that you return to this chapter periodically to update this document with the most up-to-date information about you and your wants and needs. You may also find it helpful to invite members of your support system to help you develop this plan.

Why Make a Relapse Prevention Plan?

Symptoms can interfere with our lives in a number of ways. Consider the following stories. First is Rob, describing how symptoms have impacted his relationship:

When my psychosis flares up, I start hearing this awful metallic sound. It's so distracting, and I start to think that maybe my girlfriend is somehow making that noise to bother me. I get really irritable toward her and accuse her of trying to manipulate me or torture me. I've noticed that these types of thoughts only seem to get really bad when I'm stressed out, so I'm pretty sure they're just a symptom, but in the moment, the thoughts are hard to ignore. Plus, I'm so stressed with all the noise, it's like I don't have the energy or patience to deal with anything else. It really hurts her and hurts us when we argue. I know she's built up some resentment toward me even though she's understanding. I'm worried if I can't manage this going forward, she will leave.

Notice how Annie describes how symptoms have impacted her finances:

I was diagnosed with schizoaffective disorder, bipolar type, which means I have both symptoms of schizophrenia and symptoms of bipolar disorder. My religious beliefs are very important to me and my family, but when I am in a manic episode, it's like my beliefs are taken to an extreme. My thoughts go from, It's important to help others, to I was chosen by God to help save the world. I do not need possessions to serve God. In the past, I've drained my bank account giving my savings to different charities. I've given away my laptop, my phone, even my clothes. Once the mania passed, it felt like I was left with nothing. I had to ask my family for help to get back on my feet financially.

Developing a plan of action before a crisis arises makes it easier to manage a crisis or even prevent it. Trying to develop a plan when symptoms have already gotten too distracting, too overwhelming, too frightening, or too hard is like trying to run a marathon without ever having trained for it. A well-developed relapse prevention plan can help you feel less overwhelmed, more prepared, give you more say in the care you receive, and help your support system know what you need. It is a crucial act of self-kindness and the last component of this recovery workbook.

See how Marc's relapse prevention plan has helped him avoid a cycle of rehospitalizations:

The first few years after my psychosis started felt like a roller coaster. I would be involuntarily committed for a while, discharged, and then committed again shortly thereafter for forgetting to take my meds. It didn't feel like living, just existing. The repeated hospitalizations made it impossible to keep a job. I was skeptical of the relapse prevention plan at first, but after using it for a few years, I've found it really helps me stay on track and identify when to get help before things get out of control.

Building Awareness: Think back to the recovery goals you created in chapter 2. How could reducing your risk of relapse help you achieve these goals?

_____

_____

_____

_____

_____

_____

Developing Your Plan

In the following sections, you will develop your relapse prevention plan. You will follow Rob's plan as an example.

I. About You

In the table below, write down what you notice when you are feeling good and what you notice when you are starting to feel "off". This will help you and your support system know when to intervene. The earlier you can intervene by working to reduce symptoms, the more likely you will be to avoid a mental health emergency. Here are Rob's replies:

Name: Rob		
	"When I feel good, I notice…"	**"When I don't feel good, I notice…"**
Mood	My mood fluctuates but does not feel too intense. I'm able to get out of a bad mood fairly easily by getting some rest or doing something fun.	I notice it's really hard for me to get out of a bad mood. Moods will last for days. Moods that are hardest for me are feeling angry, suspicious, or anxious.
Thoughts	I notice sounds and voices, but they aren't very distracting or loud. Voices can still be hurtful, but I remind myself that they're just thoughts and can shake them off. I notice some suspicious thoughts toward my girlfriend, but I am able to let them go.	I hear very loud noises and feel very suspicious of my girlfriend. My voices become distracting and cruel. Sometimes I think I hear other people saying disrespectful things to me, which really pisses me off. It amplifies my suspicious thoughts, and I end up not wanting to leave my room to avoid being around people.
Social Life	I get along well with my girlfriend and see my friends two or three times a week. I call or text my family every other day.	I don't respond to calls or texts as much, if at all. I have a hard time leaving the house. It feels like a lot of effort to socialize. My girlfriend and I fight often.
Substance Use	I remind myself that smoking weed makes my suspicious thoughts worse and am able to usually avoid it. I sometimes drink socially, but not often.	I smoke weed or drink every other day or daily to try to feel better.

	"When I feel good, I notice…"	"When I don't feel good, I notice…"
Hobbies and Free Time	I play in a band, and I like to make art when I have some down time. Depending on the weather, I try to get outside for at least thirty minutes a day. I feel okay being bored.	Things I used to like don't feel good or distracting enough. I go down rabbit holes online on topics that have historically been major stressors and themes in my psychosis. I get restless when I'm bored and can be impulsive.
Sleep	I generally get between seven and nine hours of sleep a night. I sleep through the night. My dreams don't bother me.	I stay up later, mostly due to anxiety. I distract myself with my phone or TV before bed, which helps me feel less anxious but disrupts my sleep. I wake up at odd times, like 3:00 a.m., and have a hard time falling back asleep. Sometimes I only sleep for four or five hours a night. My dreams can be stressful.
Appetite	I go food shopping at least once a week. My appetite is good.	Sometimes I will have suspicious thoughts about food, like I start thinking maybe it's been poisoned. These thoughts really mess up my appetite, and I end up not eating as much or having a lot of anxiety when I eat. I don't feel up to going food shopping, so I spend more money on delivery.
Work and School	I am able to work regularly. If I notice symptoms at work, I can take a break and typically feel better. I get along with my coworkers.	I have a hard time coming in. I don't feel like going, and when I do go, I feel really anxious and paranoid about my coworkers. I think they're talking about me or conspiring against me.

Environment	I've never been a super organized person, but I am able to keep up with chores, like dishes, laundry, taking out the garbage, and those types of things.	At my lowest points, when I'm really out of it, I've left food and garbage out, worn the same clothes for days, not showered... My family was really concerned. If symptoms are bad, it's really hard for me to keep up with chores. I just have too much else going on to think or care about that stuff.

Now, complete your chart. If you need more space, consider using a journal or notebook with the templates below and throughout this chapter:

Name:		
	"When I feel good, I notice…"	**"When I don't feel good, I notice…"**
Mood		
Thoughts		

	"When I feel good, I notice…"	"When I don't feel good, I notice…"
Social Life		
Substance Use		
Hobbies and Free Time		

Sleep		
Appetite		
Work and School		
Environment		

II. Things You Can Do to Stay Well

Next, identify actions you will take to proactively manage your mental health. Rob's examples are next to each category in italics.

Physical: *I will go to the grocery store once a week and focus on buying healthy snacks and things I can cook. I will go to the gym three times a week. If I don't feel like going to the gym, I will work out in my room, play basketball, or take a thirty-minute walk.*

_____

_____

_____

_____

_____

Social: *I will practice open and assertive communication with my girlfriend. I will keep in touch with my friends at least every other day and visit my family at least once a week. I will practice coping skills for my social anxiety and suspicious thoughts and schedule a night out at least once a month.*

_____

_____

_____

_____

_____

Mental: *I will take my medications as prescribed, and if I have thoughts of stopping my medications, I will talk to my psychiatrist or psychologist about it. I will practice mindfulness and relaxation coping skills for at least ten minutes a day. I will practice catching and reframing upsetting* thoughts daily. If I notice I am getting stressed, I will make an effort to reduce my responsibilities and prioritize self-care.

_____

_____

_____

_____

_____

Spiritual (This can include religious practices but can also include doing something that helps you feel connected to something larger than yourself): I will take a hike once a week so I can get some time in nature. I will keep up with my religious practices and stay involved with my religious community. I will attend peer support groups and offer to volunteer when I can.

_____

_____

_____

_____

_____

Recreational: I'll try to reduce the amount of time I am on the internet and limit my television watching to two hours a day. I will play my guitar at least four times a week. I will play with my dog at the park at least twice a week. I will work on my drawings after dinner, before bed.

_____

_____

_____

_____

_____

Environment: I'll make sure the dishes are done before going to bed. I will take the trash out when it is full. I will create a 'home' for important objects, like my keys and wallet, and make sure I am putting things back where they belong. I will clean my space at least once a week.

_____

_____

_____

_____

Responsibilities: I will go to work on time. I will challenge feelings of anxiety if my anxiety tells me I should call out or quit. I will set up auto-pay on my bills and auto-ship on my medications to make it simple. I will have a calendar showing my routine and responsibilities so I am less likely to forget them.

_____

_____

_____

_____

Remember, no one is perfect, and no one follows their routine 100 percent of the time. The most important thing is to keep trying. Do not get too down on yourself if you experience setbacks; simply make a new plan and try again.

III. Your Triggers and Warning Signs

Triggers refer to anything that may provoke a symptom. Learning more about what triggers you can help you feel more in control. For example, if you know a person, place, situation, or feeling is a trigger for you, you can prepare in advance by using a coping skill before, during, and after you encounter the trigger.

List your triggers below. Remember, a trigger can be a person, place, situation, or feeling or sensation. Refer to chapter 4 for a list of common triggers. Here are some of Rob's triggers:

Hearing loud noises, being in a crowd, fighting with my girlfriend, hearing people laughing, feeling stressed, feeling bored, feeling like people are watching me, noticing strange physical sensations, reading about stressful topics online.

Your triggers: _____

_____

_____

_____

_____

_____

_____

_____

Next, list some coping skills you can use in response to a trigger. Some of Rob's examples are below.

Trigger	Symptoms the Trigger Provokes	Coping Skill
Being in a crowd	Anxiety, suspicious thoughts, voices increase, feeling overwhelmed, increased visual hallucinations, like seeing people's faces glitch.	Practicing deep breathing, reassuring myself that I am safe, wearing sunglasses.
Fighting with my girlfriend	Anxiety, sadness, feeling shut down, sometimes feeling angry or suspicious.	Taking a break to explore my thoughts (chapter 5), reassuring myself, reframing feedback as an opportunity to improve.

Trigger	Symptoms the Trigger Provokes	Coping Skill
Hearing people laughing	Social anxiety, suspicious thoughts, voices tell me they're laughing at me.	Reassuring myself, practicing deep breathing, trying to avoid leaving the situation to build up my tolerance.

Complete the chart below with your replies. Refer to Rob's examples, above, for suggestions.

Trigger	Symptoms the Trigger Provokes	Coping Skill

While a trigger worsens symptoms *only* when you are exposed to it, warning signs refer to more pervasive changes in your mood or behavior and can be thought of as a signal that your symptoms, in general, are getting out of hand and that it is time to intervene.

Common warning signs include:

- Sleeping much less

- Noticing more grandiose, paranoid, religious, referential, or control thoughts (see chapter 5)

- Noticing voices or hallucinations are increasing or feeling more threatening

- Isolating more

- Noticing you're having trouble focusing

- Noticing changes in your self-care (for example, eating less, grooming less, trouble keeping up with chores).

Learning to identify your warning signs early can help you intervene sooner, which can reduce the likelihood of a mental health relapse or crisis.

List your warning signs below. If it helps, refer to what you brainstormed above for the "When I don't feel good, I notice…" activity. Here are some of Rob's warning signs:

1. I have trouble falling asleep for more than four nights in a row.

2. I feel less motivated and stop taking care of myself.

3. My hallucinations get louder, and voices get meaner and harder to ignore.

4. I feel more suspicious of others and isolate more. I don't talk as much to my support system and sometimes ignore their calls.

5. My family tells me I seem off or am not acting like myself.*

Your warning signs:

1. _____

2. _____

3. _____

4. _____

5. _____

6. _____

7. _____

8. _____

9. _____

10. _____

*A note about feedback from others. Sometimes symptoms can make it difficult to notice changes in our behavior. In these cases, the people we trust might be the first ones to alert us that something may be wrong. It can be hard to accept this kind of feedback, and it may be useful to remind yourself that the people in your life care about you and want the best for you. It may also be helpful to remind yourself that symptoms can distort your perception. For example, if you are feeling depressed, your thoughts are likely to be more negative and hopeless. When you are in an episode of psychosis, by nature of the symptoms themselves, you are more likely to view things differently than others. In these moments, work to reassure yourself and think of times where you were feeling and thinking differently.

Responding to warning signs. When you have noticed a warning sign, it's important to take action to reduce the likelihood of a mental health relapse. Some suggestions for actions you can take in response to a warning sign are listed below, followed by space to create your own:

- Decrease responsibilities, like taking time off work or asking for help with managing household chores.

- Ask your therapist to increase the number of sessions you have.

- Ask your psychiatric provider about medication adjustments.

- Spend more time around people you trust and feel safe with.

- Prioritize practicing coping skills more regularly.

- Increase self-care.

- Call your loved ones on the phone more often.

- Spend less time on social media.

- Go for walks in your neighborhood.

- Write your own: _____

- Write your own: _____

IV. Crisis Planning

Sometimes symptoms become so disruptive or unsafe that psychiatric hospitalization is required. Hospitals can offer you a safe place to recover, give you time to rest, and help you get connected with community resources and support. However, in our experience, many people have difficult feelings about being hospitalized. This is understandable, as hospitals can be very restrictive and include involuntary medication. You may have even felt traumatized by a prior psychiatric hospitalization. Having a say in the care you receive during an acute episode of psychosis can help reduce feelings of being powerless, frightened, or traumatized. This section is all about identifying what type of care you would like to receive during a mental health crisis.

Complete the prompts below to help your support system know what care you would like to receive during a mental health crisis.

Your care team or people you can call during a crisis:

_____

_____

_____

_____

_____

Hospitals or treatment centers you prefer:

_____

_____

_____

_____

_____

Medications that have worked for you in the past:

_____

_____

_____

_____

_____

Medications that have not worked for you in the past, and why:

_____

_____

_____

_____

_____

Coping skills that help you:

_____

_____

_____

_____

_____

Communication that works best for you (for example, giving you extra time to respond, scheduling a time to talk with you, or keeping conversations brief)**:**

_____

_____

_____

_____

_____

Signs you are feeling better (for example, sleeping more, eating more, feeling more social):

_____

_____

_____

_____

_____

A note about Behavioral Health Advance Directives. A Behavioral Health Advance Directive is a *legal document* that is similar to what you have created above. In essence, it outlines your treatment preferences in the event that you are incapacitated or unable to communicate effectively, including who will represent you during a mental health emergency, where you would like to be seen for mental health treatment, and what treatments you would like to undergo. To learn more and see if your state has an established Psychiatric Advance Directive statute, visit the National Resource Center on Psychiatric Advance Directives (http://nrc-pad.org).

V. Post-Crisis Planning and Ways Your Support System Can Help

Next, you will identify ways your support system can help you get back on your feet after a mental health crisis. It can be useful to think of a mental health crisis or relapse as similar to a physical health crisis, in that you will need additional time to rest and recover even after symptoms begin to subside. In the weeks after a mental health crisis, try to find ways to engage in self-care and delegate tasks that feel too overwhelming. Reconnect with your support system and look for people to talk with about what you have gone through. If you do not feel comfortable talking about your experiences with family or friends, consider connecting with a therapist, peer support group, or calling your local Warm Line.

Things your support system can do to help you after a crisis:

Write down some ways in which your support system could best support you after a mental health crisis.

Rob's examples: Spend more time with me at home, help me do my chores, take walks with me, make sure I am getting to my appointments on time, listen to me talk about my experience without jumping to giving me advice.

The people in your life can best support you by:

_____

_____

_____

_____

_____

_____

_____

_____

Summary

Proactive mental health care is all about taking small steps to take care of our health daily, even when our mental health feels well managed. This way, we already know what to do when symptoms start to become overwhelming. Creating a relapse prevention plan can help you feel more prepared and empowered during a mental health emergency. Keeping your plan up to date can help you and your support system best understand your needs as they change over time. Keeping a copy of your plan in an accessible location, such as in your nightstand, desk drawer, or in your wallet, will help you stay familiar with it and help friends, family, or supports find it more quickly in case of an emergency.

Final Thoughts

You've officially reached the end of *The Psychosis Workbook*! Thank you for taking the time to read our book and consider taking a moment to congratulate yourself on the hard work you have done thus far! We are honored to have been a part of your journey and hope this book has helped you feel more empowered in your recovery.

If we could leave you with one message, it would be to remember that *you are not alone*. Many people experience symptoms of psychosis to varying degrees, and support is available—though frustratingly, not nearly as available as it should be. To further address this, we compiled a list of resources, including our favorite books and websites on psychosis, which is available on the website for this book: http://www. newharbinger.com/53394. Here, you will find additional information on everything from psychosis education to a list of psychosis advocacy and peer recovery groups.

Please do not ever give up—remember that you are a worthwhile person with tremendous and unique capabilities. Our lives have certainly been enriched by the many people we have met and have had the privilege to work with through their psychosis, and we thank you for allowing us to be part of your recovery journey, too, by reading this book. We wish you all the very best as you continue on your way.

Warmly,
Laura and Jessica

Acknowledgments

To mum and dad, for always encouraging hard work, creativity, and a love for others. To Alan for twenty years of love and friendship (and probably, like, at least a few more?). To Rob, for decades of laughter. To Shannon, for embodying everything a clinician should be—on and off the job. To Cynthia and Paige, for always cheerleading my career and welcoming me home. To Mil for always being there, and to Hal for keeping him company. To R. L. and P. for joyfully accompanying me while writing this book and for giving me something to look forward to. And finally, to Jess, who introduced me to working with psychosis, mentored my dissertation, gave me a kitten, and now authored a workbook with me. I am forever grateful you decided to take this journey with me!

—Laura

Thank you to Will, for your encouragement and feedback! To Liv, for bringing me so much joy. Thank you to my parents for always supporting me. To Ron, my first supervisor in CBT for psychosis, who agreed to write our foreword! To my dear friends and family, for your acceptance and generosity. Thank you to my coworkers, who show up and work hard every single day, and to my patients, for your courage, resiliency, and inspiration. Last but not least, thank you to Laura, who made this workbook actually happen—it would still be "just a thought" if it wasn't for you.

—Jessica

References

Albers, W. M. M., D. P. K. Roeg, Y. Nijssen, I. M. B. Bongers, and J. V. Wheeghel. 2018. "Effectiveness of an Intervention for Managing Victimization Risks Related to Societal Participation for Persons with Severe Mental Illness: A Cluster RCT Study Protocol." *BMC Psychiatry* 18(1): 247.

Alberti, R., and M. Emmons. 2008. *Your Perfect Right: A Guide to Assertive Behavior*, 9th ed. San Luis Obispo, CA: Impact Press.

Alemon, A., T. M. Lincoln, R. Bruggerman, I. Melle, J. Arends, C. Arongo, and H. Knegtering. 2017. "Treatment of Negative Symptoms: Where Do We Stand, and Where Do We Go?" *Schizophrenia Research* 186: 55–62.

Bailey, A. 2022. "What Selena Gomez Shared About Her Psychotic Episode, Living with Bipolar, and Overcoming Suicidal Thoughts." *Elle*, November 4. https://www.elle.com/culture/celebrities/a41871246/selena-gomez-my -mind-and-me-psychotic-episode.

Barrantes-Vidal, N. 2004. "Creativity and Madness Revisited from Current Psychological Perspectives." *Journal of Consciousness Studies* 11(3–4): 58–78.

Beck, A. T. 1979. *Cognitive Therapy of Depression*. New York: Guilford Press.

Bellack, A. S., and A. Drapalski. 2012. "Issues and Developments on the Consumer Recovery Construct." *World Psychiatry* 11(3): 156–160.

Belli, S. R. 2009. "A Psychobiographical Analysis of Brian Douglas Wilson: Creativity, Drugs, and Models of Schizophrenic and Affective Disorders." *Personality and Individual Differences* 46(8): 809–819.

Bennett, S. S., and P. Indman. 2019. *Beyond the Blues: Understanding and Treating Prenatal and Postpartum Depression and Anxiety*. San Francisco: Untreed Reads.

Bentall, R. 2024. "Delusional Beliefs and the Madness of Crowds." In *Decoding Delusions: A Clinician's Guide to Working with Delusions and Other Extreme Beliefs*, edited by K. V. Hardy and D. Turkington. Washington DC: American Psychiatric Association.

Berk, M. S., G. R. Henriques, D. M. Warman, G. K. Brown, and A. T. Beck. 2004. "A Cognitive Therapy Intervention for Suicide Attempters: An Overview of the Treatment and Case Examples." *Cognitive and Behavioral Practice* 11: 265–277.

Blake, P., A. A. Collins, and M. V. Seeman. 2015. *Women and Psychosis: An Information Guide*. Toronto: Centre for Addiction and Mental Health.

Blumer, M. 2002. "The Illness of Vincent van Gogh." *American Journal of Psychiatry* 159: 519–526.

Bobes, J., C. Arango, M. Garcia-Garcia, and J. Rejas. 2010. "Prevalence of Negative Symptoms in Outpatients with Schizophrenia Spectrum Disorders Treated with Antipsychotics in Routine Clinical Practice: Findings from the CLAMORS Study." *Journal of Clinical Psychiatry* 71(3): 280–286.

Bordoloi, M., and U. Ramtekkar. 2018. "Relationship Between Sleep and Psychosis in the Pediatric Population: A Brief Review." *Medical Sciences* 6(3): 76.

Bornheimer, L. A., N. Tarrier, A. P. Brinen, J. Li, M. Dwyer, and J. A. Himle. 2021. "Longitudinal Predictors of Stigma in First-Episode Psychosis: Mediating Effects of Depression." *Early Intervention in Psychiatry* 15(2): 263–270.

Bowie, C. R., and P. D. Harvey. 2006. "Cognitive Deficits and Functional Outcome in Schizophrenia." *Neuropsychiatric Disease and Treatment* 2(4): 531–536.

Brohan, E., and G. Thornicroft. 2010. "Stigma and Discrimination of Mental Health Problems: Workplace Implications." *Occupational Medicine* 60: 414–420.

Capaldi, C. A., R. L. Dopko, and J. M. Zelenski. 2014. "The Relationship Between Nature Connectedness and Happiness: A Meta-Analysis." *Frontiers in Psychology* 5.

Carretti, B., E. Borella, and R. De Beni. 2007. "Does Strategic Memory Training Improve the Working Memory Performance of Younger and Older Adults?" *Experimental Psychology* 54(4): 311–320.

Cicerone, K. D., Y. Goldin, K. Ganci, A. Rosenbaum, J. V. Wethe, D. M. Langenbahn, J. F. Malec, et al. 2019. "Evidence-Based Cognitive Rehabilitation: Systematic Review of the Literature from 2009 Through 2014." *Archives of Physical Medicine and Rehabilitation* 100(8): 1515–1533.

Compton, M. T., and B. Broussard. 2009. *The First Episode of Psychosis: A Guide for Patients and Their Families.* New York: Oxford University Press.

Correll, C. U., and N. R. Schooler. 2020. "Negative Symptoms in Schizophrenia: A Review and Clinical Guide for Recognition, Assessment, and Treatment. *Neuropsychiatric Disease and Treatment* 16: 519–534.

Dalai Lama and D. Tutu. 2001. *An Open Heart: Practicing Compassion in Everyday Life.* Boston: Little, Brown.

Doran, G. T. 1981. "There's a SMART Way to Write Management's Goals and Objectives." *Journal of Management Review* 70: 35–36.

Eigen, M. 2005. *Psychotic Core.* London: Karnac.

Ellett, L. 2023. "Mindfulness for Psychosis: Current Evidence, Unanswered Questions, and Future Directions." *Psychology and Psychotherapy: Theory, Research, and Practice* 1–7.

Eskenazi, G. 1998. "Lionel Aldridge, 56, Stalwart on Defense for Packer Teams." *New York Times*, February 14. Gale Academic OneFile. https://link.gale.com/apps/doc/A150229251/AONE?u=anon~ffc03e22&sid=google Scholar&xid=c1322827.

Fellinger, M., T. Waldhoer, D. Konig, B. Hinterbuchinger, N. Pruckner, J. Baumgartner, S. Vyssoki, and B. Vyssoki. 2019. "Seasonality in Bipolar Disorder: Effect of Sex and Age." *Journal of Affective Disorders* 243: 322–326.

Firth, J. R., P. Carney, R. French, J. Elliott, J. Cotter, and A. R. Young. 2018. "Long-Term Maintenance and Effects of Exercise in Early Psychosis." *Early Intervention in Psychiatry* 12: 578–585.

Firth, J., J. Cotter, R. Elliott, P. French, and A. Yung. 2015. "A Systematic Review and Meta-Analysis of Exercise Interventions in Schizophrenia Patients." *Psychological Medicine* 45: 1343–1361.

Foreman, S. S. 1954. "Psychosis of Famous Men." Master's Thesis, June 30. Eastern Illinois University, 20–21.

Freeman, D., T. Brugha, H. Meltzer, R. Jenkins, D. Stahl, and P. Bebbington. 2010. "Persecutory Ideation and Insomnia: Findings from the Second British National Survey of Psychiatric Morbidity." *Journal of Psychiatric Research* 44(15):1021–1026.

Frith, C. D. 1992. *The Cognitive Neuropsychology of Schizophrenia.* Mahwah, NJ: Lawrence Erlbaum.

Geoffroy, P. A., F. Bellivier, J. Scott, C. Boudebesse, M. Lajnef, S. Gard, J. P. Kahn, et al. 2013. "Bipolar Disorder with Seasonal Pattern: Clinical Characteristics and Gender Influences." *Chronobiology International* 30(9): 1101–1107.

Grant, P. M., and A. T. Beck. 2009. "Defeatist Beliefs as a Mediator of Cognitive Impairment, Negative Symptoms, and Functioning in Shizophenia." *Schizophrenia Bulletin* 35(4): 798–806.

Grover, L. E., R. Jones, N. J. Bass, and A. McQuillin. 2022. "The Differential Associations of Positive and Negative Symptoms with Suicidality." *Schizophrenia Research* 248: 42–49.

Guo, X., J. Zhai, Z. Liu, M. Fang, B. Wang, C. Wang, B. Hu, et al. 2010. "Effect of Antipsychotic Medication Alone versus Combined with Psychosocial Intervention on Outcomes of Early-Stage Schizophrenia: A Randomized One-Year Study." *Archives of General Psychiatry* 67(9): 895–904.

Haddad, P. M., and C. U. Correll. 2018. "The Acute Efficacy of Antipsychotics in Schizophrenia: A Review of Recent Meta-Analyses." *Therapeutic Advances in Psychopharmacology* 8(11): 303–318.

Harvey, P. D., D. Koren, A. Reichenberg, and C. Bowie. 2006. "Negative Symptoms and Cognitive Deficits: What Is the Nature of Their Relationship?" *Schizophrenia Bulletin* 32(2): 250–258.

Hayes, S. C., K. D. Strosahl, and K. G. Wilson. 2012. *Acceptance and Commitment Therapy: The Process and Practice of Mindful Change*, 2nd ed. New York: Guilford Press.

Ho, B. C., P. Nopoulos, M. Flaum, S. Arndt, and N. C. Andreasen. 1988. "Two-Year Outcome in First-Episode Schizophrenia: Predictive Value of Symptoms for Quality of Life." *American Journal of Psychiatry* 155: 1196–1201.

Hogarty, G. E., and R. F. Ulrich. 1998. "The Limited Effects of Antipsychotic Medication on Schizophrenia Relapse and Adjustment and the Contributions of Psychosocial Treatment." *Journal of Psychiatric Research* 32(3–4): 243–250.

Huang, Z., Y. Guo, Y. Ruan, S. Sun, T. Lin, J. Ye, J. Li, et al. 2020. "Associations of Lifestyle Factors with Cognition in Community-Dwelling Adults Aged 50 and Older: A Longitudinal Cohort Study." *Frontiers of Aging in Neuroscience* 12: 601487.

Hunter, C. L., J. L. Goodie, M. S. Oordt, and A. C. Dobmeyer. 2015. *Integrated Behavioral Health in Primary Care*. Washington, DC: American Psychological Association.

Jablensky, A., N. Sartorius, G. Ernberg, M. Anker, A. Korten, J. E. Cooper, R. Day, and A. Bertelsen. 1992. "Schizophrenia: Manifestations, Incidence, and Course in Different Cultures. A World Health Organization Ten-Country Study." *Psychological Medicine Monograph Supplement* 20: 1–97.

Jordan, G., K. MacDonald, M. A. Pope, E. Schorr, A. K. Malla, and S. N. Iyer. 2018. "Psychosis Changes Experienced After a First Episode of Psychosis: A Systematic Review." *Psychiatric Services* 69(1): 84–99.

Jose, J., and M. M. Joseph. 2018. "Imagery: It's Effects and Benefits on Sports Performance and Psychological Variables: A Review Study." *International Journal of Physiology, Nutrition and Physical Education* 3(2): 190–193.

Kendler, K. S. 2020. "The Development of Kraepelin's Concept of Dementia Praecox: A Close Reading of Relevant Texts." *JAMA Psychiatry* 77(11): 1181–1187.

Kessler, R. C., S. Aguilar-Gaxiola, J. Alonso, S. Chatterji, S. Lee, and T. B. Ustun. 2009. "The WHO World Mental Health (WMH) Surveys." *Psychiatrie* 6(1): 5–9.

Linehan, M. M. 2015. *DBT Skills Training Manual*, 2nd ed. New York: Guilford Press.

Luther, L., G. M. Coffin, R. L. Firmin, K. A. Bonfils, K. S. Minor, and M. P. Salyers. 2016. "A Test of the Cognitive Model of Negative Symptoms: Associations Between Defeatist Performance Beliefs, Self-Efficacy Beliefs, and Negative Symptoms in a Non-Clinical Sample." *Psychiatry Research* 269: 278–285.

Mancuso, F., W. P. Horan, R. S. Kern, and M. F. Green. 2011. "Social Cognition in Psychosis: Multidimensional Structure, Clinical Correlates, and Relationship with Functional Outcome." *Schizophrenia Research* 125(2–3): 143–151.

Mamalaki, E., S. Charisis, C. A. Anastasiou, E. Ntanasi, K. Georgiadi, V. Balomenos, M. H. Kosmidis, et al. 2022. "The Longitudinal Association of Lifestyle with Cognitive Health and Dementia Risk: Findings from the HELIAD Study." *Nutrients* 14(14): 2818.

Martinez, A., V. Huddy, and R. Bentall. 2024. "The Psychology of Paranoid Beliefs." In *Decoding Delusions: A Clinician's Guide to Working with Delusions and Other Extreme Beliefs*, edited by Kate Hardy and Douglas Turkington. Washington, DC: American Psychiatric Association Publishing.

McCarthy-Jones, S. 2012. *Hearing Voices: The Histories, Causes and Meanings of Auditory Verbal Hallucinations*. Cambridge, UK: Cambridge University Press.

McCarthy-Jones, S., A. Waegeli, and J. Watkins. 2013. "Spirituality and Hearing Voices: Considering the Relation." *Psychosis* 5(3): 247–258.

McGrath, J. J., S. Saha, A. Al-Hamzawi, J. Alonso, E. J. Bromet, R. Bruffaerts, J. M. Caldas-de-Almeida, et al. 2015. "Psychotic Experiences in the General Population: A Cross-National Analysis Based on 31,261 Respondents from 18 Countries." *JAMA Psychiatry* 72(7): 697–705.

Menditto, A. A., N. C. Beck, P. Stuve, J. A. Fisher, M. Stacy, M. B. Logue, and L. J. Baldwin. 1996. "Effectiveness of Clozapine and a Social Learning Program for Severely Disabled Psychiatric Inpatients." *Psychiatric Services* 47(1): 46–51.

Mojtabai, R., R. A. Nicholson, and B. N. Carpenter. 1998. "Role of Psychosocial Treatments in Management of Schizophrenia: A Meta-Analytic Review of Controlled Outcome Studies." *Schizophrenia Bulletin* 24(4): 569–587.

National Alliance of Mental Illness (NAMI). 2024. "About Mental Illness." https://www.nami.org/About-Mental-Illness.

Neff, K. n.d. "Exercise 3. Exploring Self-Compassion though Writing." *Self-Compassion*. https://self-compassion.org/exercise-3-exploring-self-compassion-writing.

Norris, C. J., D. Creem, R. Hendler, and H. Kober. 2018. "Brief Mindfulness Meditation Improves Attention in Novices: Evidence from ERPs and Moderation by Neuroticism." *Frontiers of Human Neuroscience* 12: 315.

Palaniyappan, L., V. Balain, J. Radua, and P. F. Liddle. 2012. "Structural Correlates of Auditory Hallucinations in Schizophrenia: A Meta-Analysis." *Schizophrenia Research* 137: 169–173.

Pillny, M., B. Schlier, and T. M. Lincoln. 2020. "'I Just Don't Look Forward to Anything.' How Anticipatory Pleasure and Negative Beliefs Contribute to Goal-Directed Activity in Patients with Negative Symptoms of Psychosis." *Schizophrenia Research* 222: 429–436.

Posner, M. I., M. K. Rothbart, and Y. Tang. 2015. "Enhancing Attention Through Training." *Current Opinion in Behavioral Sciences* 4: 1–5.

Rabinowitz, J., S. Z. Levine, G. Garibaldi, D. Bugarski-Kirola, C. G. Berardo, and S. Kapur. 2012. "Negative Symptoms Have Greater Impact on Functioning Than Positive Symptoms in Schizophrenia: Analysis of CATIE Data." *Schizophrenia Research* 137: 147–150.

Ramsey, D. 2021. *Eat to Beat Depression and Anxiety Nourish Your Way to Better Mental Health in Six Weeks.* New York: HarperCollins.

Sánchez-Izquierdo, M., and R. Fernández-Ballesteros. 2021. "Cognition in Healthy Aging." *International Journal of Environmental Research and Public Health* 18(3): 962.

Schildkrout, B. 2017. "Joan of Arc—Hearing Voices." *The American Journal of Psychiatry* 174(12): 1153–1154.

Sharma, I., J. Srivastava, A. Kumar, and R. Sharma. 2016. "Cognitive Remediation Therapy for Older Adults." *Journal of Geriatric Mental Health* 3(1): 57–65.

Sheffield, J. M., N. R. Karcher, and D. M. Barch. 2018. "Cognitive Deficits in Psychotic Disorders: A Lifespan Perspective." *Neuropsycholy Review* 28: 509–533.

Sheffield, J. M., L. E. Williams, J. U. Blackford, and S. Heckers. 2013. "Childhood Sexual Abuse Increases Risk of Auditory Hallucinations in Psychotic Disorders." *Comprehensive Psychiatry* 54(7): 1098–1104.

Sher, L., M. A. Oquendo, and J. J. Mann. 2001. "Risk of Suicide in Mood Disorders." *Clinical Neuroscience Research* 1(5): 337–344.

Spaulding, W. D., S. M. Silverstein, and A. A. Menditto. 2017. *The Schizophrenia Spectrum,* 2nd ed. Boston: Hogrefe Publishing Corporation.

Stanley, B., and G. Brown. 2012. "Safety Planning Intervention: A Brief Intervention to Mitigate Suicide Risk." *Cognitive and Behavioral Practice* 19(2): 256–264.

Strong, T., and N. R. Pyle. 2009. "Constructing a Conversational 'Miracle': Examining the 'Miracle Question' as It Is Used in Therapeutic Dialogue." *Journal of Constructivist Psychology* 22(4): 328–353.

Substance Abuse and Mental Health Services Administration. 2021. "The NSDUH Report." Rockville, MD: Office of Applied Studies.

Tang, Y., R. Tang, and M. I. Posner. 2016. "Mindfulness Meditation Improves Emotional Regulation and Reduces Drug Abuse." *Drug and Alcohol Dependence* 163: S13–S18.

Taylor, S. E. 2011. "Social Support: A Review." In *The Oxford Handbook of Health Psychology*, edited by H. S. Friedman. Oxford, UK: Oxford University Press.

Tondo, L., G. H. Vazquez, and R. J. Baldessarini. 2010. "Mania Associated with Antidepressant Treatment: Comprehensive Meta-Analytic Review." *Acta Psychiatrica Scandinavia* 121: 404–314.

Turkington, D., D. Kingdon, S. Rathod, S. K. J. Wilcock, A. Brabban, P. Cromarty, R. Dudley, et al. 2009. *Back to Life, Back to Normality: Volume 1: Cognitive Therapy, Recovery, and Psychosis*. Cambridge, UK: Cambridge University Press.

Turkington, D., and H. M. Spencer, eds. 2019. *Back to Life, Back to Normality. Volume 2, CBT Informed Recovery for Families with Relatives with Schizophrenia and Other Psychoses*. New York: Cambridge University Press.

US Department of Health and Human Services. 2018. *Physical Activity Guideline for Americans*, 2nd ed. Washington, DC: US Department of Health and Human Services.

van der Tuin, S., S. H. Booij, A. J. Oldehinkel, D. van den Berg, J. T. W. Wigman, U. Lang, and I. Kelleher. 2023. "The Dynamic Relationship Between Sleep and Psychotic Experiences Across the Early Stages of the Psychosis Continuum." *Psychological Medicine* 53: 7646–7654.

Varese, F., F. Smeets, M. Drukker, R. Lieverse, T. Lataster, W. Vietchtbauer, J. Read, J. van Os, and R. P. Bentall. 2012. "Childhood Adversities Increase the Risk of Psychosis: A Meta-Analysis of Patient-Control, Prospective- and Cross-Sectional Cohort Studies." *Schizophrenia Bulletin* 38(4): 661–671.

Vartanian, G. V., B. Y. Li, A. P. Chervenak, O. J. Walch, W. Pack, P. Ala-Laurila, and K. Y. Wong. 2015. "Melatonin Suppression by Light in Humans Is More Sensitive Than Previously Reported." *Journal of Biological Rhythms* 30(4): 351–354.

Vilhauer, R. P. 2017. "Stigma and Need for Care in Individuals Who Hear Voices." *International Journal of Social Psychiatry* 63(1): 5–13.

Volpato, E., C. Cavalera, G. Gastelnuovo, E. Molinari, and F. Pagnini. 2022. "The 'Common' Experience of Voice-Hearing and Its Relationship with Shame and Guilt: A Systematic Review." *BMC Psychiatry* 22: 281.

Winton-Brown, T. T., P. Fusar-Poli, M. A. Ungless, and O. D. Howes. 2014. "Dopaminergic Basis of Salience Dysregulation in Psychosis." *Trends in Neurosciences* 37(2): 85–94.

Wood, L., R. Byrne, E. Burke, G. Enache, and A. P. Morrison. 2017. "The Impact of Stigma on Emotional Distress and Recovery from Psychosis: The Mediatory Role of Internalized Shame and Self-Esteem." *Psychiatry Research* 255: 94–100.

Wood, L., R. Byrne, G. Enache, and A. P. Morrison. 2018. "Acute Inpatients' Experiences of Stigma from Psychosis: A Qualitative Exploration." *Stigma and Health* 3(1): 1.

World Health Organization. 2022. "Mental Disorders." https://www.who.int/news-room/fact-sheets/detail/mental-disorders.

Wykes, T., and W. D. Spaulding. 2011. "Thinking About the Future of Cognitive Remediation Therapy—What Works and Could We Do Better?" *Schizophrenia Bulletin* 37(2): S80–S90.

Xu, Z., M. Müller, K. Heekeren, A. Theodoridou, D. Dvorsky, S. Metzler, A. Brabban, et al. 2016. "Self-Labelling and Stigma as Predictors of Attitudes Towards Help-Seeking Among People at Risk of Psychosis: 1-Year Follow-Up." *European Archives of Psychiatry and Clinical Neuroscience* 266: 79–82.

Yaribeygi, H., Y. Panahi, H. Sahraei, T. P. Johnston, and A. Sahebkar. 2017. "The Impact of Stress on Body Function: A Review." *EXCLI Journal* 16: 1057–1072.

Yates, K., U. Lang, M. Cederlof, F. Boland, P. Taylor, M. Cannon, F. McNicholas, J. DeVylder, and I. Kelleher. 2019. "Association of Psychotic Experiences with Subsequent Risk of Suicidal Ideation, Suicide Attempts, and Suicide Deaths." *JAMA Psychiatry* 76(2): 180–189.

Laura Dewhirst, PsyD, is a licensed clinical psychologist who focused her predoctoral and postdoctoral training on the treatment of more persistent mental health concerns, including personality disorders, bipolar disorders, co-occurring substance use disorders, and behavioral concerns. She has specialized training in the treatment of schizophrenia spectrum disorders and psychosis, and has served this population in inpatient, residential, and outpatient settings across the United States.

Jessica Murakami-Brundage, PhD, is a licensed clinical psychologist who has over twenty years of experience working with individuals with serious mental illness (SMI). She is passionate about the recovery model and has served on the American Psychological Association (APA) Task Force for Serious Mental Illness and Severe Emotional Disturbance (TFSMI/SED), as well as APA's SMI Psychology Specialty Council.

Foreword writer **Ron Unger, LCSW**, is a therapist who specializes in cognitive behavioral therapy (CBT) for the treatment of psychosis.

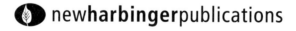

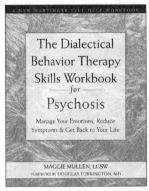
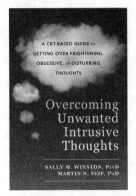
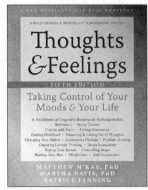
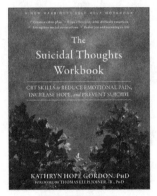
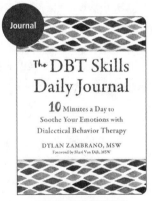
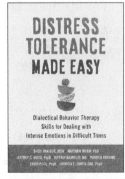

Did you know there are **free tools** you can download for this book?

Free tools are things like **worksheets, guided meditation exercises**, and **more** that will help you get the most out of your book.

You can download free tools for this book—whether you bought or borrowed it, in any format, from any source—from the New Harbinger website. All you need is a NewHarbinger.com account. Just use the URL provided in this book to view the free tools that are available for it. Then, click on the "download" button for the free tool you want, and follow the prompts that appear to log in to your NewHarbinger.com account and download the material.

You can also save the free tools for this book to your **Free Tools Library** so you can access them again anytime, just by logging in to your account! Just look for this button on the book's free tools page. ➡ **+ Save this to my free tools library**

If you need help accessing or downloading free tools, visit **newharbinger.com/faq** or contact us at **customerservice@newharbinger.com**.